W9-BSA-194

Pathophysiology, Evaluation and Management of Valvular Heart Diseases

Sponsored by
Weill Medical College of Cornell University, and
The New York Cardiological Society of the American College of Cardiology, New York State Chapter

Publication made possible by unrestricted grants from
Johnson and Johnson, Inc., and
The Howard L. and Judie Ganek Philanthropic Fund of the Jewish Communal Fund

Advances in Cardiology

Vol. 39

Series Editor

Jeffrey S. Borer *New York, N.Y.*

KARGER

Pathophysiology, Evaluation and Management of Valvular Heart Diseases

Developed from "Valves in the Heart of the Big Apple: Evaluation and Management of Valvular Heart Diseases" May 10–12, 2001, New York, N.Y.

A Conference Organized by The Howard Gilman Institute for Valvular Heart Diseases, Weill Medical College of Cornell University

Volume Editors

Jeffrey S. Borer *New York, N.Y.*
O. Wayne Isom *New York, N.Y.*

58 figures and 43 tables, 2002

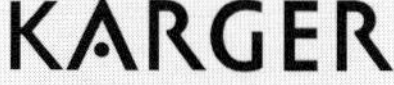

Basel · Freiburg · Paris · London · New York ·
New Delhi · Bangkok · Singapore · Tokyo · Sydney

Advances in Cardiology

Jeffrey S. Borer, MD
Gladys and Roland Harriman Professor of Cardiovascular Medicine
Chief, Division of Cardiovascular Pathophysiology
Co-Director, The Howard Gilman Institute for Valvular Heart Diseases
Weill Medical College
Cornell University
New York, NY 10021 (USA)

Library of Congress Cataloging-in-Publication Data

Pathophysiology, evaluation and management of valvular heart disease / volume editors, Jeffrey S. Borer, O. Wayne Isom.
p. ; cm. – (Advances in cardiology, ISSN 0065-2326 ; v. 39)
Developed from "Valves in the heart of the big apple; evaluation and management of valvular heart diseases, May 10–12, 2001, New York, N.Y. A conference organized by the Howard Gilman Institute for Valvular Heart Diseases, Weill Medical College of Cornell University."
Includes bibliographical references and index.
ISBN 3805574029 (hard cover : alk. paper)
1. Heart valves–Diseases–Pathophysiology. 2. Heart valves–Diseases–Surgery. I. Borer, J. S. (Jeffrey S.) II. Isom, O. Wayne. III. Cornell University. Howard Gilman Institute for Valvular Heart Diseases. IV. Series.
[DNLM: 1. Heart Valve Diseases–therapy–Congresses 2. Aortic Valve–physiopathology–Congresses. 3. Heart Valve Diseases–surgery–Congresses. 4. Mitral Valve–physiopathology–Congresses. WG 260 P297 2002]
RC681.A25 A38 vol. 39 RC685.V2
616.1′2 s–dc21
[616.1′2507] 2002016277

Bibliographic Indices. This publication is listed in bibliographic services, including Current Contents® and Index Medicus.

Drug Dosage. The authors and the publisher have exerted every effort to ensure that drug selection and dosage set forth in this text are in accord with current recommendations and practice at the time of publication. However, in view of ongoing research, changes in government regulations, and the constant flow of information relating to drug therapy and drug reactions, the reader is urged to check the package insert for each drug for any change in indications and dosage and for added warnings and precautions. This is particularly important when the recommended agent is a new and/or infrequently employed drug.

www.karger.com
Printed in Switzerland on acid-free paper by Reinhardt Druck, Basel
ISSN 0065–2326
ISBN 3–8055–7402–9

Contents

Introduction

Diseased heart valves are a growing public health concern. As death due to coronary artery disease and to non-cardiac causes has been shifted to increasingly older age groups or partially eliminated, valvular diseases have been recognized as common and progressive concomitants of aging. This is particularly true in the USA, Canada and Western Europe, where the prevalence of acquired rheumatic valvular diseases in the first three decades of life has diminished markedly compared with 50 or more years ago. However, the increasing prevalence of valvular diseases also is apparent in other parts of the world, where rheumatic fever remains a very important problem. In addition, modern diagnostic modalities and epidemiological research have led to increasing recognition of the impact of hereditary metabolic predispositions, nonfatal coronary/ischemic events and progression of congenital lesions that are clinically inapparent at birth on the total burden of valvular diseases in the aging population. The result is a growing expenditure of healthcare resources for managing clinical sequelae of dysfunctional heart valves. Consequently, recurring examination is appropriate to define current knowledge of valvular disease pathophysiology, epidemiology, natural history and management strategies. This volume represents one such examination.

More than 25 years ago, at separate institutions, we began research in valvular diseases in conjunction with management of patients with these disorders. Over the course of more than a quarter century of our own experience and that of colleagues throughout the world, it has become increasingly clear that the pathophysiology of valvular diseases varies widely with the affected valve, the specific hemodynamic characteristics of the lesion and the nature of any associated cardiovascular pathology and that, consequently, each major valve disease category requires individualized attention both from researchers and from clinicians. At Weill Medical College of Cornell University, our joint efforts in exploring concepts and evaluating patients with heart valve diseases ultimately led to the creation of The Howard Gilman Institute for Valvular Heart Diseases. The Institute has allowed us to focus intensively on the pathophysiology and management of valvular diseases in an environment characterized by progressively increasing prevalence and complexity of these diseases. The conference entitled, '*Valves in the Heart of the Big Apple: Evaluation and Management of Valvular Heart Diseases*', organized by the Institute and jointly sponsored by The Weill Medical College of Cornell University and The New York Cardiological Society of the American College of Cardiology, New York State Chapter, represents one manifestation of that focus. This publication is drawn from the presentations of several faculty members who participated in the first convocation of that conference, on May 10–12, 2001. The articles were prepared and updated after the conference to provide succinct statements of important contemporary concepts and concerns. In addition to relating current thinking about appropriate timing of surgery for patients with various valve lesions (always a moving target as evaluation strategies become more precise and therapies become more effective and safe), sections of this volume discuss specific technical issues regarding evolving surgical approaches and selected pathophysiological considerations at the systemic, whole organ, cellular and molecular levels. The latter two areas increasingly are appropriate and timely foci of investigation as the cardiology/ cardiac surgery community works toward meaningful enhancement of prognostic strategies and development of novel pharmacotherapy, and even molecular therapy, to beneficially alter the most fundamental pathophysiology of these diseases before, during and after surgery.

We would like to thank the faculty members that produced the articles for this volume and to acknowledge that each of them was importantly involved, by virtue of his or her own research, in creating the new knowledge about which each has written. In addition, we would like to thank The Howard Gilman Foundation, which supports much of the research at our Institute and which enabled organization of '*Valves in the Heart of the Big Apple*' and this volume, Johnson & Johnson, Inc., which provided a much appreciated unrestricted educational grant enabling preparation of articles for this publication, and the Howard L. and Judie Ganek Philanthropic Fund of the Jewish Communal Fund, which provided an unrestricted grant to cover publication costs. Our appreciation also extends to the providers of unrestricted educational support for the conference: in addition to our primary benefactor, Johnson & Johnson, Inc., these included Edwards Life Science, American Home Products-Wyeth-Ayerst Laboratories, Medtronic, Otsuka America Pharmaceutical, Inc., St. Jude Medical, Sulzer Carbomedics/

Scanlon Cardiopulmonary, Pfizer, Inc., Astra Zeneca Pharmaceuticals, Sankyo Pharma, and Pfizer.

We believe this volume represents a useful adjunct for clinician and researcher. We hope readers will agree.

Jeffrey S. Borer, MD
O. Wayne Isom, MD

Borer JS, Isom OW (eds): Pathophysiology, Evaluation and Management of Valvular Heart Diseases.
Adv Cardiol. Basel, Karger, 2002, vol 39, pp 1–6

The Epidemiology of Valvular Heart Disease: An Emerging Public Health Problem

Phyllis G. Supino, Jeffrey S. Borer, Andrew Yin

Division of Cardiovascular Pathophysiology and The Howard Gilman Institute for Valvular Heart Diseases, Weill Medical College of Cornell University, New York, N.Y., USA

Valvular heart diseases (VHD), both regurgitant and stenotic, are the most predictable causes of heart failure [1]. Quantitatively, though far less prevalent than coronary artery disease, valvular diseases are among the more important underlying causes of heart failure and of sudden death [1–3]. Though the mitral (M) and aortic (A) valves are most frequently affected, the tricuspid (T) and pulmonic (P) valves also can be dysfunctional.

For many years, the prevalence of VHD in our society was underestimated. However, introduction of the echocardiogram and its increasingly widespread use has indicated a remarkably high proportion of patients with asymptomatic valve disease [4–6] that can be expected to progress to clinical importance at a relatively slow but predictable rate. Epidemiological studies, using noninvasive imaging as well as clinical evaluation, indicate that VHD generally follows a prolonged course from hemodynamically mild inception to later hemodynamic severity, and another relatively long interval from hemodynamic severity to clinical debility or death [7]. As intercurrent causes of death and debility diminish and therapeutic options for VHD are progressively developed and perfected, this population increasingly becomes a target for potentially life-enhancing and life-prolonging intervention.

The population at risk can be expected to increase over time. Several reports have chronicled the resurgence of acute rheumatic fever and associated valve-related sequelae in the USA during the past few decades [8–11]. Nonetheless, current etiologic surveys indicate that VHD now results far more commonly from genetically determined characteristics than from the immunologic sequelae of a distant infection or from infection itself [12, 13]. When inherited factors result in VHD, clinically important dysfunction generally does not appear until after the age of procreation. Therefore, there is no selective disadvantage for reproduction among individuals carrying predisposing traits. Consequently, progressive increase in VHD prevalence can be expected as the population increases.

Indeed, the apparent magnitude of VHD prevalence, its projected increase and its potential sequelae justify the claim that VHD represents a burgeoning public health problem. However, the extent of this problem remains unclear. Though several published studies have estimated the prevalence and or incidence of VHD, these evaluations have been performed in fundamentally different populations that have been relatively small [14–17] and/or highly circumscribed [4–6, 18–20], and have produced widely varying estimates from which extrapolation may be inaccurate.

To obtain a larger sampling frame for estimating the distribution of various forms of valve disease and to add to existing knowledge about the impact of VHD on the utilization of healthcare resources, we recently undertook a longitudinal study of VHD-associated hospitalizations over a 17-year interval in New York State. Our objectives were to review temporal trends in hospitalization rates and invasive procedures among inpatients with a diagnosis of AV, MV, TV and/or PV HD and to compare these rates according to type of disease, demographic factors, and etiology. Preliminary results of this analysis are presented in this paper.

Methods

Data for this study were derived from New York's 'State-Wide Planning and Research Cooperative System' inpatient database, or SPARCS [21]. SPARCS is a comprehensive, integrated computer-based archive comprising information for each discharge from over 250 nonfederal acute care facilities throughout New York State, abstracted from medical records by trained hospital-based personnel. Age, gender, race, year and month of discharge, principal and secondary diagnoses, and principal and secondary procedures are included, the latter recorded according to the ICD-9 classification system. SPARCS is designed to provide the incidence of conditions requiring hospitalizations. Therefore, the unit of analysis is the case rather than the individual patient.

Our analysis spans the period from 1983 through 1999, i.e., from the first year in which reliable SPARCS data were consistently available, through the last year for which complete records were obtainable. We analyzed all records with either principal or secondary ICD-9 codes reflecting isolated diseases of the MV and/or AV, TV and PV. However, for this preliminary analysis, subject identifiers were not employed. No attempt was made to distinguish between principal and secondary diagnoses since these are highly dependent on the individual coder and hospital. For comparison, we also examined trends in the total number of hospitalizations in New York State during this period.

Linear regression analysis was employed to model temporal trends in demographics and in other variables of interest (including number of hospitalizations and number of therapeutic valve procedures (open chest valvotomy or other valve repair, valve replacement or percutaneous balloon valvuloplasty)) for the entire population and selected subgroups.

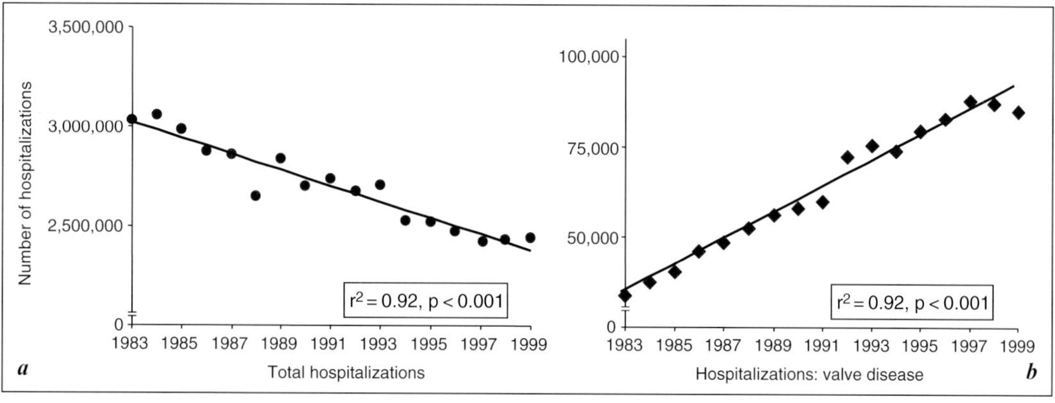

Fig. 1. Temporal changes in number of hospitalizations in New York State between 1983 and 1999: (***a***) total number of hospitalizations (all causes) vs. (***b***) hospitalizations including a valvular heart disease diagnosis (mitral, aortic, tricuspid and/or pulmonic valve diseases).

Results

Characteristics of the Patient Population

In total, over 1 million cases met our inclusion criteria. Of these, approximately 40% were hospitalized with VHD during the last 5 years (average age 65 years at hospital discharge or death). The majority was white and female, though the ratio of females to males, non-whites to whites, and average age at hospitalization increased sharply over the 17-year study interval ($p < 0.001$, both variables). Most patients either had isolated AV or MV HD. Etiology was believed to be rheumatic in a fifth of hospitalizations.

Temporal Changes in Hospitalizations

Though hospitalizations in New York State decreased approximately 20% from 1983 to 1999 ($p < 0.001$, fig. 1a), the incidence of hospitalizations including a diagnosis of VHD increased almost 3-fold during this period ($p < 0.001$, fig. 1b). The rate of increase in mitral stenosis (MS) and/or insufficiency (MR) was more than double than that observed for aortic stenosis (AS) and/or insufficiency (AR). Though far fewer in number, directionally similar changes were seen for TV and PV diseases. Rheumatic VHD, alone, also was associated with progressively more hospitalizations during the 17-year interval, though the rate of increase nominally was lower than for total VHD and, thus, for nonrheumatic VHD. Rheumatic disease distribution also was different than nonrheumatic: as might be expected, the most common isolated valve disorder in this population was MS.

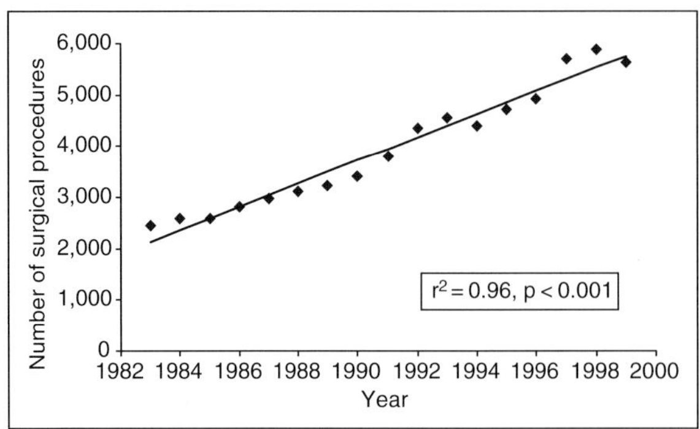

Fig. 2. Temporal change in number of therapeutic valve procedures performed between 1983 and 1999. Procedures include open chest valvotomy or other valve repair, valve replacement and percutaneous balloon valvuloplasty.

Performance of Therapeutic Valve Procedures

Therapeutic valve procedures (predominantly valve replacements) also increased linearly between 1983 and 1999 ($p < 0.001$), both for all patients with VHD and for the subgroup with VHD of rheumatic etiology (fig. 2). The performance of these procedures increased with the age of the patient throughout the entire range of ages represented. Though females predominated in the cohort, males were more likely to undergo valve surgery, a pattern that intensified over time. When white patients were compared with non-white patients, no racial disparities were found. Certainly, these dramatic increases reflect improvements in surgical techniques during the study interval, allowing application of these treatments to a wider population and, to a lesser extent, from more accurate clinical identification of patients at risk. Nonetheless, at least in part, the numbers also reflect the increase in patients at risk.

Conclusions

Several factors limit our ability to infer true prevalence rates from the SPARCS data. First, SPARCS data are case- or incidence-based, rather than patient-based. Until we add the subject identifiers, it is not possible to exclude multiple hospitalizations in the same patient. Nonetheless, particularly in recent years when these numbers are the largest, Medicare reimbursement rules would tend to limit multiple hospitalizations for the same problem in the same year. Second, the data presented here do not include outpatient visits for VHD. Outpatient visits are likely to reflect the largest component of medical visits and undoubtedly involve many patients who have not been hospitalized. These facts would tend to cause our data to underestimate, perhaps substantially, the true prevalence of VHD in the population. Third, since cases were selected on the basis of diagnosis, it is not possible to determine whether the observed temporal patterns are due to improved recognition by clinicians or to more illness in the population. Addition of patient identifiers will resolve this problem. Nonetheless, the data clearly indicate that the incidence of hospitalization and surgical treatment for VHD is increasing. The trends we observed are so marked and so prolonged that it is also reasonable to conclude that the increase in VHD-related hospitalizations will continue to rise as the population increases. Second, though not responsible for the majority of cases, rheumatic fever contributes substantially to the development of VHD, perhaps due to immigration of previously affected or susceptible individuals or to an increase in rheumatic fever in the USA. The data suggest that the prevalence of rheumatic etiologies also will continue to increase until more effective measures are initiated globally to prevent rheumatic fever. Finally, despite the limitations noted above, analysis of the SPARCS data strongly suggest that inferences drawn from small cross-sectional population studies generally are correct, that is, that valvular abnormalities are present in a large proportion of our population, that they are hemodynamically important in a far smaller but still substantial portion and that, increasingly, health care resources must be targeted to dealing with this predictable cause of heart failure.

Acknowledgements

The authors wish to acknowledge Srilatha Atluri, BS, for her prodigious efforts in data compilation and presentation and in facilitating statistical analysis.

Dr. Borer is supported in part as The Gladys and Roland Harriman Professor of Cardiovascular Diseases (Gladys and Roland Harriman Foundation, New York, N.Y.). In addition, this work was supported in part by an unrestricted grant from The Howard Gilman Foundation (New York, N.Y.), and by grants from the Ronald and Jean Schiavone Foundation, White House Station, N.J., the Charles and Jean Brunie Foundation, Bronxville, N.Y., the Mary A.H. Rumsey Foundation, New York, N.Y., the Irving A. Hansen Foundation, New York, N.Y., The David Margolis Foundation, New York, N.Y., the Howard L. and Judie Ganek Philanthropic Fund of the Jewish Communal Fund, New York, N.Y., the Messinger Family Foundation, New York, N.Y., and by a much appreciated gift from Stephen and Suzanne Weiss, Greenwich, Conn.

References

1 Wilson PW: An epidemiologic perspective of systemic hypertension, ischemic heart disease, and heart failure. Am J Cardiol 1997;80:3J–8J.

2 Mangion JR, Tighe DA: Aortic valvular disease in adults. A potentially lethal clinical problem. Postgrad Med 1995;98:127–135, 140.

3 Grigioni F, Enriquez-Sarano M, Ling LH, Bailey KR, Seward JB, Tajik AJ, Frye RL: Sudden death in mitral regurgitation due to flail leaflet. J Am Coll Cardiol 1999;34:2086–2087.
4 Reid CL, Gardin JM, Yunis C, Kurosaki T, Flack JM: Prevalence and clinical correlates of aortic and mitral regurgitation: The Cardia Study. Circulation 1994;90:I–282.
5 Singh JP, Evans JC, Levy D, Larson MG, Freed LA, Fuller DL, Lehman B, Benjamin EJ: Prevalence and clinical determinants of mitral, tricuspid, and aortic regurgitation (The Framingham Heart Study). Am J Cardiol 1999;83:897–902.
6 Jones EC, Devereux RB, Roman MJ, Liu JE, Fishman D, Lee ET, Welty TK, Fabsitz RR, Howard BV: Prevalence and correlates of mitral regurgitation in a population-based sample (The Strong Heart Study). Am J Cardiol 2001;87:298–304.
7 Follman DF: Aortic regurgitation: Identifying and treating acute and chronic disease. Postgrad Med 1993;93:83–90.
8 Wesdake RM, Graham TP, Edward KM: An outbreak of acute rheumatic fever in Tennessee. Pediatr Infect Dis J 1990;9:97–100.
9 Griffiths SP: Acute rheumatic fever in New York City (1969–1988): A comparative study of two decades. J Pediatr 1990;116:882–887.
10 Ayoub EM: Resurgence of rheumatic fever in the United States. The changing picture of a preventable illness. Postgrad Med 1992;92:133–136, 139–142.
11 Feldman T: Rheumatic mitral stenosis. On the rise again. Postgrad Med 1993;93:93–94, 99–104.
12 Hochreiter C, Niles N, Devereux RB, Kligfield P, Borer JS: Mitral regurgitation: Relationship of right and left ventricular performance to clinical and hemodynamic findings and to prognosis in medically and surgically treated patients. Circulation 1986;73:900–912.
13 Borer JS, Hochreiter C, Herrold EM, Supino P, Krieger K, Isom OW: Prediction of indications for valve replacement among asymptomatic or minimally symptomatic patients with chronic aortic regurgitation and normal left ventricular performance. Circulation 1998;97:525–534.
14 Kostucki W, Wandenbossche JL, Friart A, Englert M: Pulsed Doppler regurgitant flow patterns of normal valves. Am J Cardiol 1986;309–313.
15 Akasaka T, Yoshikawa J, Yoshida K, Okumachi F, Koizumi K, Shiratori K, Takao S, Shakudo M, Kato H: Age-related valvular regurgitation: A study by pulsed Doppler echocardiography. Circulation 1987;76:262–265.
16 Berger M, Hecht SR, Van Tosh A, Lingam U: Pulsed and continuous wave Doppler of assessment of valvular regurgitation in normal subjects. J Am Coll Cardiol 1989;13:1540–1545.
17 Brand A, Dollberg S, Keren A: The prevalence of valvular regurgitation in children with structurally normal hearts: A color Doppler echocardiographic study. Am Heart J 1992;123:177–180.
18 Samanek M, Slavik Z, Zborilova B, Hrobonova V, Voriskova M, Skovranek J: Prevalence, treatment, and outcome of heart disease in live-born children: A prospective analysis of 91,823 live-born children. Pediatr Cardiol 1989;10:205–211.
19 Lindroos M, Kupari M, Heikkilä, Tilvis R: Prevalence of aortic valve abnormalities in the elderly: An echocardiographic study of a random population sample. J Am Coll Cardiol 1993;21: 1220–1225.
20 Stewart BF, Siscovick D, Lind BK, Gardin JM, Gottdiener JS, Smith VE, Kitzman DW, Otto CM: Clinical factors associated with calcific aortic valve disease. J Am Coll Cardiol 1997;29:630–634.
21 Quan JM: SPARCS: The New York State Health Care Data System. J Clin Comput 1980;8:255–263.

Jeffrey S. Borer, MD, Division of Cardiovascular Pathophysiology/The Howard Gilman Institute for Valvular Heart Diseases, Weill Medical College of Cornell University, The New York-Presbyterian Hospital New York Weill Cornell Medical Center, 525 East 68th Street, New York, NY 10021 (USA)

Borer JS, Isom OW (eds): Pathophysiology, Evaluation and Management of Valvular Heart Diseases.
Adv Cardiol. Basel, Karger, 2002, vol 39, pp 7–14

The Cellular and Molecular Basis of Heart Failure in Regurgitant Valvular Diseases: The Myocardial Extracellular Matrix as a Building Block for Future Therapy

Jeffrey S. Borer, Sharada L. Truter, Edmund McM. Herrold, Phyllis G. Supino, John N. Carter, Anuj Gupta

Division of Cardiovascular Pathophysiology, Department of Cardiothoracic Surgery and The Howard Gilman Institute for Valvular Heart Diseases, Weill Medical College of Cornell University, New York, N.Y., USA

Volume loading from hemodynamically severe aortic and/or mitral regurgitation (AR, MR) cannot be substantially reversed with currently available medications. Maintenance of blood pressures compatible with consciousness and activity when upright requires limitation of the doses of vasodilator drugs such that diminution of regurgitant flow can be no more than modest to moderate. Valve replacement or repair must be employed to completely obliterate regurgitant flow. Therefore, surgical therapy is the most effective approach for relief of congestive heart failure (CHF) from valvular regurgitation. Surgery also is effective in preventing CHF development. However, the short-term risks and long-term effects of operation on myocardial function require that valve surgery should be withheld until objective evidence indicates that the risk of not operating exceeds that of performing surgery.

Evidence of prognostically important risk differs in asymptomatic patients with AR and MR. For patients with AR, this evidence includes (1) subnormal left ventricular (LV) ejection fraction (EF) at rest, (2) relatively marked LV dilatation at rest and (3) substantially subnormal intrinsic contractility, which can be determined from radionuclide cineangiographic LVEF change from rest to exercise (ΔLVEF) modified by echocardiographic LV afterload, measured as end-systolic stress (ESS) [1]. The latter is of particular interest because of the pathophysiological implications of the relation of intrinsic contractility to outcome. For patients with MR, progression to CHF and death also is predicted by indices of myocardial performance and contractility. Empirically, these include LVEF that falls below a value 10% above the lower limit of the nominally normal range [2], the presence of subnormal right ventricular (RV) EF at rest [3] (almost always associated with supernormal pulmonary artery pressures [3]) and, perhaps, a fall in RVEF from rest to exercise [4], suggesting subnormal RV contractile reserve. Progression also is predicted by the development of atrial fibrillation, which may be indirectly related to cardiac mechanics.

The relation of outcome and contractility suggests the potential for therapeutic intervention to prevent myocardial decompensation. Pharmacological interventions of an earlier era, focused directly on the contractile machinery, have not demonstrated morbidity-preventing or life-prolonging efficacy. However, interventions aimed at the fundamental pathobiology, including the alterations in myocardial cell biology and molecular controls caused by volume loading, might be expected to provide such benefits. New approaches to therapy at the cellular and molecular levels require new knowledge of the fundamental pathophysiology of CHF in regurgitant valvular diseases.

Evidence Linking Contractility and Outcome

The relation between contractility and outcome has been demonstrated best in patients with AR, a setting in which contractility can be measured relatively easily by noninvasive means. (Contractility measurement in MR is complicated by ambiguity in the determination of end-systole owing to differences in timing of the closure of the aortic valve and cessation of mitral regurgitation and LV mechanical contraction.) Since the cellular and molecular data presented later in this article relate specifically to AR, contractility data will be presented only for this lesion. Contractility has been closely related to outcome in AR using a noninvasive index of contractility [1]. In a population of 104 largely asymptomatic patients with normal LVEF at rest and severe AR that was followed for an average of 8 years and a maximum of 15 years, the contractility index was significantly better related to subsequent outcome than was any other functional or geometric measure. Contractility was determined as ΔLVEF adjusted for change in ESS from rest to exercise. When the population was divided arbitrarily into terciles based on contractility at study outset, the tercile with the best contractility had only a 1.8% annual progression rate to CHF while the tercile with the poorest contractility (though manifesting normal LVEF at rest) had a 10-fold greater rate of progression; the middle tercile manifested outcome incidence approximately midway between the polar extremes.

Extracellular Matrix Biology and Contractility Loss

A clue to the potential importance of the myocardial extracellular matrix (ECM) in mediating contractility loss in chronic AR was reported a decade ago with the definition of the time course of LVEF recovery after aortic valve replacement (AVR) for AR [5]. Earlier reports of postoperative recovery were importantly impacted by the relatively rudimentary intraoperative myocardial preservation methods used in many centers until 20 years ago; results of these early studies suggested little or no improvement in LVEF after AVR. In contrast, application of modern myocardial preservation methods is associated with relatively marked postoperative improvement in LVEF compared with preoperative values. However, maximal recovery is achieved gradually over the course of 3 years after AVR [5]. On average, LVEF at rest reaches a plateau (generally well within the normal range) approximately 2 years after operation, while LVEF during exercise (which almost invariably is lower than the resting value prior to operation) continues to improve during an additional year, surpassing the resting value before reaching its plateau. These findings indicate prolonged, extensive LV remodeling, reversing an even more prolonged pathologic remodeling process during the chronic volume overload state. Elucidation of underlying cellular and molecular processes should provide many targets for therapeutic alteration to slow or prevent pathophysiologically important facets of the response to volume overload that leads to CHF.

LV mass increases rapidly during the month after induction of experimental AR. During the first week, hypertrophy is driven primarily by supernormal synthesis rates both of total myocardial protein and of contractile proteins [6]. Later, as the process approaches chronicity, myocardial protein degradation rates fall progressively below normal while synthesis rates fall to normal or even mildly subnormal levels. Reduction of degradation rates predominates; therefore, subnormal total and contractile protein degradation rates then drive continuing hypertrophy [6]. Preliminary kinetic studies in experimental MR suggest similar results. Thus, the disordered cell biology of AR and MR features disruption of the metabolic kinetics of myocyte-derived contractile proteins. However, this process is unlikely to account for the slow recovery of LV function after AVR, or for loss of LV function prior to operation. The reason is that the half-lives of the contractile proteins are sufficiently short so that, if only contractile proteins were involved in the remodeling process, the heart would have been reconstructed more than 100 times during the 3 years required for maximal recovery of rest and exercise LVEF.

A more plausible candidate process to account for prolonged remodeling was elucidated by histological observations in the animals manifesting disordered contractile protein kinetics. These studies revealed myocardial fibrosis, often severe [7]. ECM proteins, comprising the fibrotic lesions, have relatively long half-lives, better matched to remodeling duration. Quantitative analysis indicated that mild to moderate fibrosis accompanied myocyte hypertrophy even when hemodynamically severe AR was 'compensated', i.e., when CHF had not supervened. In animals with CHF, fibrosis invariably was particularly exuberant. Animals in the CHF subcohort also evidenced myocyte degradation, though AR was no more severe than in the compensated group [7]. However, despite myocytolysis and associated fibrosis, no inflammatory infiltrate was observed. Thus, it is likely that fibrosis was a primary response to LV dilatation, not a secondary response to myocyte destruction. Several processes might then account for myocytolysis: mechanical alteration of blood flow or cell shape by fibrosis, apoptosis, or some other, less well-characterized mechanism.

Fibrotic lesions primarily comprise fibroblasts and their secretory products, the ECM proteins. Though less voluminous than cardiomyocytes, fibroblasts are more numerous and, in fact, represent the predominant cell line in the myocardium. The primary product of the fibroblast is collagen. However, the fibroblast also synthesizes many non-collagen, glucosamine-containing proteins that appear to have specific physiological functions and potential pathophysiological importance when their production or structure are altered. Normally, fibroblasts and ECM form the scaffold that configures the relation between myocardial cellular and vascular elements. Fibrosis, featuring excessive myocardial ECM, may contribute importantly to disordered contractility in AR. A pathophysiological role of fibrosis is suggested by the physical link observed between the cardiomyocyte cytoskeleton and the ECM. This bond appears to be affected by specific proteins, including dystrophins and related peptides, that pierce the sarcolemma [8]. The physical relation between myocyte and matrix appears to mediate and be necessary for normal contractile force. Experimental evidence suggests that the glucosamine-containing ECM protein, fibronectin, may mediate binding to integrins, facilitating the myocyte-matrix interaction [9].

ECM alterations caused by AR have been evaluated in cultures of cardiac fibroblasts isolated from rabbits with chronic experimental AR and from normal rabbits. In the animals from which the fibroblast cultures were created, AR varied from mild to severe as judged by echocardiographic regurgitant fraction. Differential display PCR and selective subtractive hybridization revealed abnormal expression of 8 genes by AR fibroblasts [10, 11], some upregulated and some downregulated. The physiological and potential pathophysiological roles of each of these abnormally expressed genes are poorly understood. However, the likely importance of 3 of the 8 is relatively unambiguous. These 3 code for ECM proteins [10], none of them collagen isoforms and all glucosamine-containing; each gene is upregulated in AR, suggesting a disproportion of these proteins relative to that seen in the ECM of the normal heart. Most prominent among them was fibronectin. To determine whether the abnormal gene expression is translated to abnormal protein synthesis, two corollary studies were performed. The first study compared ECM incorporation of tritiated proline, a collagen component, and of tritiated glucosamine, a component of non-collagen ECM glycoproteins like fibronectin, by cardiac fibroblasts cultured from AR and normal hearts [10]. Though proline incorporation was statistically indistinguishable between normal and AR fibroblast cultures, glucosamine incorporation by AR fibroblasts was twice normal. Then, protein synthesis was specifically evaluated with Western blots for two common collagen ECM isoforms and for fibronectin (as a prototype of the non-collagen ECM proteins) and by gelatin-sepharose affinity chromatography, an assay method highly specific for fibronectin. Collagen synthesis by AR fibroblasts was no different than normal [10]. In contrast, fibronectin synthesis was upregulated in AR cultures by a ratio averaging approximately 2:1. Preliminary data from a parallel study indicate that activity of metalloprotease MMP-2, an enzyme that degrades myocardial collagen, is increased by AR, while fibronectinase activity is unaffected [12], and that AR fibroblasts produce an autocrine factor that can stimulate normal cardiac fibroblasts to reproduce the ECM synthesis pattern usually resulting from AR [unpubl. observation].

These data indicate that matrix biology is disordered in AR hearts but they do not resolve the sequence of the disorder and, therefore, the likely causal events. To test the hypothesis that was generated by the histopathological findings, that selective hyperproduction of fibronectin and other non-collagen matrix elements is a primary response to the volume loading of AR rather than secondary responses to myocyte injury and inflammation, cultures of normal cardiac fibroblasts were created during application of biaxial mechanical strain. The strain values were based on a previously validated mathematical model describing LV stress and strain patterns as a function of volume and pressure throughout the cardiac cycle [13]. The primary culture of each cell line was divided into three subcultures, one to which no strain was applied (control), one in which strain values mimicked those of the normal LV at midwall (control) and one in which the applied strain modeled that measured at LV midwall in chronic, severe AR; strain was applied cyclically, 60 times per minute [10,14], to reproduce the effect of the normal heart rate. Relative to unstrained cultures or cultures to which strains of the normal LV were applied, cultures facing AR strains manifest proline and glucosamine incorporation, ECM protein synthesis pattern and gene expression changes that closely paralleled those observed in cultures of fibroblasts from hearts with AR in vivo when they were compared with fibroblasts from normal hearts [10, 14]. Therefore, ECM remodeling in AR must result, at least in part, as a primary response to the mechanical stresses of volume loading [10].

This observation also identifies as potential therapeutic targets the elements of the pathway that transduces abnormal mechanical strain to the production of ECM that is disproportionately rich in glucosamine-containing proteins. Selective modulation of myocardial fibrosis has not yet been achieved. However, nonselective pharmacologic modulation in AR is possible, as demonstrated by the effects of the quinalone derivative, vesnarinone, in suppressing cardiac fibroblast survival [15]. Importantly, this intervention appears to feature a substantial therapeutic advantage: fibroblast survival is suppressed at doses an order of magnitude lower than those used clinically (and causing excessive and potentially lethal cardiac arrhythmias) and at doses 10-fold higher in normal cardiac fibroblast cultures than in AR fibroblasts [15]. Selective modulation will require precise definition of mechanical stress-to-gene expression pathway responsible for production of pathophysiologically important ECM. The relevant pathway in AR fibroblasts is not known, but we have demonstrated that AR upregulates a reaction that normally is the last step prior to activation of a fibronectin promoter [16]. This step involves activation of Jun kinase, leading to phosphorylative activation of the promoter. We are now studying the effect of AR on the reaction that precedes Jun kinase activation in other systems, that is, activation of a mitogen-activated kinase kinase, MEK 4/7; preliminary unpublished data suggest that this step also is upregulated in AR. Moving backward through the known pathway will permit identification of all reactions that are involved in the transduction of mechanical stresses. If a reaction in this pathway does not respond to AR, an appropriate alternative can be sought that is relevant for AR. Ultimately, the initial mechanical response element that initiates the pathway can be defined. This approach will identify multiple targets for potentially therapeutic intervention, either with conventional drugs or with genetic material and, simultaneously, will elucidate multiple descriptors that can be measured to refine prognostication.

In summary, in the setting of volume overload from AR and, possibly, from other parallel conditions, mechanical alterations and resulting wall stresses directly affect cardiac fibroblast biology resulting in production of ECM featuring abnormal proportions of normal components. The remodeled ECM is relatively rich in glucosamine-containing proteins that are likely to affect myocyte-matrix interaction, potentially modulating contractility. In its early stages, this process may be a compensatory adaptation with beneficial effects. When prolonged and progressive, it may compromise ventricular mechanical function and lead to heart failure. Selective suppression of this process may be useful in preventing or reversing heart failure in regurgitant valvular diseases. Additionally, the understanding of ECM biology gained from studies in AR may be useful in retarding CHF development in ischemic heart disease, in which noninfarcted LV myocardium faces mechanical stresses similar to those of AR.

Acknowledgements

Dr. Borer is the Gladys and Roland Harriman Professor of Cardiovascular Medicine at Cornell and was supported in part during this work by an endowment from the Gladys and Roland Harriman Foundation, New York, N.Y. In addition, the work reported herein was supported in part by National Heart Lung and Blood Institute, Bethesda, Md. (RO1-HL-26504), and by grants from The Howard Gilman Foundation, New York, N.Y., The Schiavone Family Foundation, White House Station, N.J., The Charles and Jean Brunie Foundation, Bronxville, N.Y., The David Margolis Foundation, New York, N.Y., The American Cardio-Vascular Research Foundation, New York, N.Y., The Irving A. Hansen Foundation, New York, N.Y., The Mary A.H. Rumsey Foundation, New York, N.Y., The Messinger Family Foundation, New York, N.Y., the Daniel and Elaine Sargent Charitable Trust, New York, N.Y., the A.C. Israel Foundation, Greenwich, Conn., and by much appreciated gifts from Maryjane and the late William Voute, Bronxville, N.Y., and Stephen and Suzanne Weiss, Greenwich, Conn.

References

1 Borer JS, Hochreiter C, Herrold EM, Supino P, Aschermann M, Wencker D, Devereux RB, Roman MJ, Szulc M, Kligfield P, Isom OW: Prediction of indications for valve replacement among asymptomatic or minimally symptomatic patients with chronic aortic regurgitation and normal left ventricular performance. Circulation 1998;97:525–534.

2 Enriquez-Sarano M, Tajik AJ, Schaff HV, Orszulak TA, Bailey KR, Frye RL: Echocardiographic prediction of survival after surgical correction of organic mitral regurgitation. Circulation 1994; 90:830–837.

3 Hochreiter C, Niles N, Devereux RB, Kligfield P, Borer JS: Mitral regurgitation: Relationship of non-invasive descriptors of right and left ventricular performance to clinical and hemodynamic findings and to prognosis in medically and surgically treated patients. Circulation 1986;73: 900–912.

4 Rosen S, Borer JS, Hochreiter C, Supino P, Roman MJ, Devereux RB, Kligfield P, Bucek J: Natural history of the asymptomatic/minimally symptomatic patient with severe mitral regurgitation secondary to mitral valve prolapse and normal right and left ventricular performance. Am J Cardiol 1994;74:374–380.

5 Borer JS, Herrold EM, Hochreiter C, Roman MJ, Supino P, Devereux RB, Kligfield P, Nawaz H: Natural history of left ventricular performance at rest and during exercise after aortic valve replacement for aortic regurgitation. Circulation 1991;84(suppl III):133–139.

6 Magid NM, Borer JS, Young MS, Wallerson DC, Demonteiro C: Suppression of protein degradation in the progressive cardiac hypertrophy of chronic aortic regurgitation. Circulation 1993;87: 1249–1257.

7 Liu SK, Magid NM, Fox PR, Goldfine SM, Borer JS: Fibrosis, myocyte degeneration and heart failure in chronic experimental aortic regurgitation. Cardiology 1998;90:101–109.

8 Leiden J: The genetics of dilated cardiomyopathy – Emerging clues to the puzzle. N Engl J Med 1997;337:1080–1081.

9 Ahumada G, Saffitz J: Fibronectin in the rat heart: Link between cardiac myocytes and collagen. J Histochem Cytochem 1984;32:383–388.

10 Borer JS, Truter SL, Herrold EM, Falcone DJ, Pena M, Dumlao T, Lee J, Supino PG: Myocardial fibrosis in chronic aortic regurgitation: molecular and cellular response to volume overload. Circulation 2002, in press.

11 Truter SL, Goldin D, Kolesar J, Dumlao TF, Borer JS: Abnormal gene expression of cardiac fibroblasts in experimental aortic regurgitation. Am J Ther 2000;7:237–243.

12 Truter SL, Lee JA, Dumlao TF, Young K, Borer JS: Collagenase activity selectively increases in aortic regurgitation to suppress collagen content in fibrosis. J Am Coll Cardiol 2001;37:2: 1047–107:473A.
13 Herrold EM, Carter JN, Borer JS: Volume-overload-related shape change limits mass increase with wall thickening but only minimally reduces wall stress. Computers in Cardiology, 1992; IEEE Publ 0276-6547/92:287–290.
14 Herrold EM, Borer JS, Truter SL, Carter JN, Liu F, Dumlao TF: Myocardial fibrosis in aortic regurgitation: Fibroblast response to in vitro strain is magnitude dependent. Circulation 2000; 102(suppl II):530.
15 Ross JS, Goldfine SM, Herrold EM, Borer JS: Differential response to vesnarinone by cardiac fibroblasts isolated from normal and aortic regurgitant hearts. Am J Ther 1998;5:369–375.
16 Truter SL, Lee JA, Dumlao TF, Borer JS: Increased fibronectin expression in aortic regurgitation: Role of stress activated protein kinase/c-Jun NH2-terminal kinase pathway. J Am Coll Cardiol 2001;37:2:875.3:487A.

Jeffrey S. Borer, MD, The Division of Cardiovascular Pathophysiology,
The New York-Presbyterian Hospital New York Weill Cornell Center, 525 East 68th Street,
New York, NY 10021 (USA)

Borer JS, Isom OW (eds): Pathophysiology, Evaluation and Management of Valvular Heart Diseases.
Adv Cardiol. Basel, Karger, 2002, vol 39, pp 15–24

Emerging Biology of Mitral Regurgitation: Implications for Further Therapy

Mark R. Starling

University of Michigan and VA Ann Arbor Healthcare Systems,
Ann Arbor, Mich., USA

This paper will take you into the world of myocardial contractility, neurohumoral system modeling and gene expression. These areas are somewhat different from those presented elsewhere in this volume, but these concepts will dovetail smoothly with them. The studies described herein were predicated on the concept that there must be a pathobiologic process that is stimulated in the volume overload state, which gradually and reversibly affects myocardial performance. This must be so because, based on our understanding of the natural history of mitral regurgitation (MR), the myocardium cannot be transformed rapidly from functioning normally to being irreversibly impaired, since there is no specific and definable incident that would affect such a dramatic change in myocardial performance. Rather, there must be a gradual transition from normal contractility to impaired contractility.

Initial Observations

Based on this premise, it was hypothesized early in our work that myocardial contractility may indeed be impaired early in the natural history of MR when left ventricular (LV) pump performance, e.g. ejection fraction (EF), remains normal. This concept was tested in a large group of normal subjects and patients with MR, who remained in normal sinus rhythm and had no definable coronary artery disease. The average LVEF in the normal subjects was approximately 61%, while that in the MR patients averaged 60%. Although there was a wide range of

LVEF in the MR patients, only a small number of those patients had truly subnormal LVEF. In contrast, the vast majority of the MR patients had impaired contractility, when contractility was assessed using the elastance concept and confirmed using complex myocardial stiffness calculations [1–3].

Interestingly, in those MR patients who had a normal preoperative LVEF but impaired contractility, there was a unique response to successful mitral valve surgery [1]. As expected, the LV end-diastolic volume indices fell dramatically with relief of the volume overload and, then, increased slightly at 1 year. There was also a decline in LV end-systolic volume by 3 months, which remained reduced at 1 year. As a consequence, LVEF declined early following mitral valve surgery, many into the subnormal range, but there was recovery of LV pump performance in the majority of these patients to well within the normal range at 1 year. Although some of this recovery of LV ejection performance appeared to be related to remodeling of the LV over time, the possibility that the preoperative contractile impairment was reversible remained untested.

Accordingly, in a subgroup of these patients, who had preoperative contractile studies, 1 year postoperative contractile studies were also performed [4]. These studies indicated that in several of the MR patients with impaired contractility prior to mitral valve surgery, contractile performance recovered to normal following successful mitral valve surgery. These patients could be identified by certain preoperative characteristics, including an LV end-systolic volume index that averaged 44 ml/m^2 compared to 86 ml/m^2 in those whose contractility remained impaired. These observations raised the question of the underlying pathobiology of contractile impairment in the volume overload state of MR and why this was potentially reversible.

Control of Contractility

If one examines the hypothesized control of contractility in the intact circulation, there are three contributors [5]. The dominant contributor is the β-adrenergic receptor system stimulated by the sympathetic nervous system, which directly modulates contractility and indirectly modulates contractility through the force-frequency relationship. The force-frequency relationship, itself, can modulate contractile performance directly over a wide range of heart rates. Finally, length-dependent activation of contractile performance also is a contributor, though its effect is relatively minor compared to the other two control systems.

In an elegant study using epicardial muscle strips from donor hearts and patients with MR, Mulieri et al. [6] demonstrated that the force-frequency relationship was dramatically impaired in MR patients. While peak isometric tension increased progressively up to a stimulation frequency of approximately

150–160 beats per minute in the normal donor hearts, it was flattened if not negative in the muscle strips from the MR patients. This impaired force-frequency relationship in the MR patients could be partially reversed by the administration of forskolin to the muscle bath, which directly stimulates the β-adrenergic receptor system. This provided strong evidence for an impaired force-frequency relationship and raised the issue of whether the β-adrenergic receptor system played a major role in the impaired force-frequency relationship. Whether the β-adrenergic receptor system directly contributed to impaired contractility in the intact circulation in patients with MR remained untested.

Unifying Hypothesis

To test this concept, we proposed a unifying hypothesis, which is reflected in the old adage, 'MR begets more MR'. As regurgitant volume increases, it impinges upon forward stroke volume, which must be augmented to maintain effective tissue perfusion. Therefore, compensatory mechanisms, including preload reserve and sympathetic nervous system activity, are called upon to maintain adequate stroke volume. If the sympathetic nervous system is activated, particularly over a long period of time, alterations in β-adrenergic receptor responsivity may occur and lead through their modulation of contractility to impaired myocardial performance.

Sympathetic Nervous System Activity

To test whether the sympathetic nervous system is activated in MR patients, we used a complex modeling approach, based strongly in the physiology concepts of the sympathetic nervous system [7]. Sympathetic nerve terminals reside in the extravascular space, which is not accessible. Norepinephrine (NE) is released from the nerve terminal. Most is taken back up into the nerve terminal, metabolized, or sequestered in vesicles for re-release. Some NE traverses the neuroeffector junction and stimulates an effector cell; other NE is transferred from the extravascular space into the vascular space; yet other NE present in the vascular space may move into the extravascular space where it stimulates the effector cell or is taken up into the nerve terminal. This is a complex system. Prior studies have looked at the sympathetic nervous system in numerous ways, but they have not attempted to model this system to obtain NE secretion rates in the extravascular space, a more proximate index of sympathetic nervous system activity, or to obtain a more complete understanding of this complex physiologic system.

To model this system, we used [^{3}H]-NE infusions (fig. 1) and arterial blood sampling to assess the systemic sympathetic nervous system and blood sampling

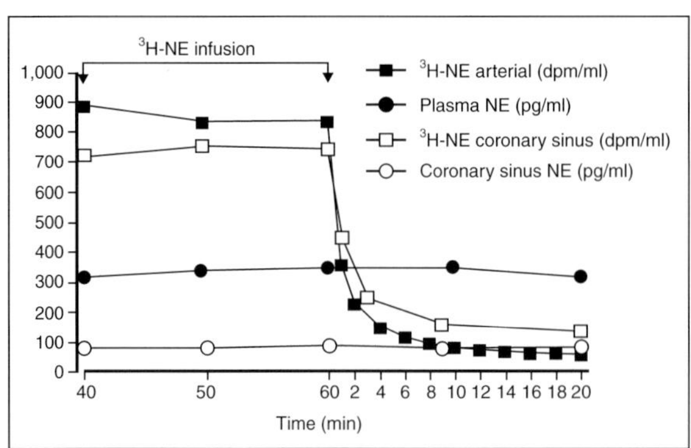

Fig. 1. The [^{3}H]-norepinephrine (NE) kinetic study protocol is shown for both the systemic and organ-specific cardiac sympathetic nervous system activity assessment. Note that following 60 min of [^{3}H]-NE infusion, there is steady state both in the systemic arterial and coronary sinus circulations, and there is no effect on endogenous NE levels. Following completion of the infusion, there is a nonlinear decay in [^{3}H]-NE in both the systemic arterial and coronary sinus circulations, which is minimally fit by a bi-exponential, suggesting that a two-compartmental model would best fit these data.

from the coronary sinus to assess organ-specific cardiac sympathetic nervous activity. When [^{3}H]-NE level reaches steady state and the infusion is discontinued, there is a rapid bi-exponential decay. This suggests that the minimum model that would effectively provide kinetic information regarding the sympathetic nervous system is a two-compartment model. This is consistent both for the systemic and organ-specific cardiac sympathetic nervous systems. From this model (fig. 2), we can calculate the components of systemic sympathetic nervous system activity, i.e., NE secretion rates (NE_2), as well as metabolic clearance rates, transfer constants, volumes of distribution, etc.

These calculations indicated that, in comparison to control subjects, patients with MR had increased NE secretion rates. In contrast, the NE transfer constants from the extravascular space into the vascular space were higher for the control subjects compared to the patients with MR. This suggests that the re-uptake function of NE into the nerve terminal in the MR patients was more active. Thus, one might conclude that the sympathetic nerve terminals in the MR patients were releasing more NE but also re-accumulating NE more rapidly compared to control subjects. This suggests a very active sympathetic nervous system, which we would not have been able to characterize without the model.

When these NE secretion rates were related to functional parameters, there were several interesting observations. First, those MR patients who had more advanced clinical symptomatology had higher NE secretion rates than those who were asymptomatic or minimally symptomatic. Similarly, NE secretion

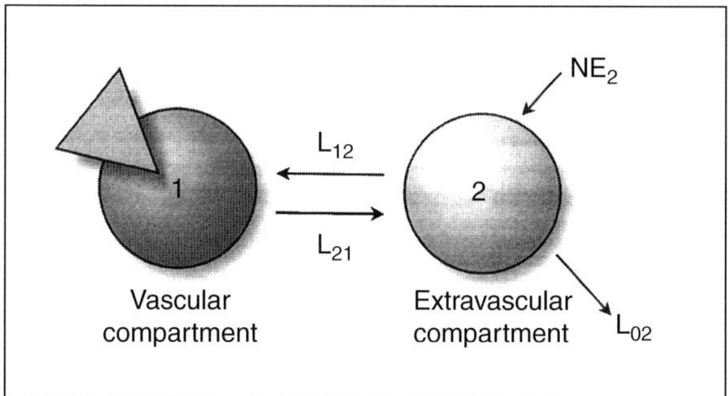

Fig. 2. The model developed by Linares et al. [7] is graphically illustrated. Compartment 1 represents the vascular space and can be sampled, while compartment 2 represents the extravascular space, which cannot be sampled but into which norepinephrine (NE) is secreted. The more proximate index of sympathetic nervous system activity, NE_2, represents NE secretion rates into the extravascular space, and it is but one index that can be obtained from the modeling system to more completely understand the complexities of the sympathetic nervous system at the systemic or organ-specific level. Additional parameters include metabolic clearance rates, transfer constants both into and out of the extravascular space, as well as volumes of distribution. While NE levels are simple to obtain from venous blood sampling, they are determined by a complex interplay, which not only includes the parameters described in the two-compartment model, but also regional blood flow and extraction across the regional vascular bed, among others. Thus, the two-compartment modeling system provides a more physiologically relevant index of the secretion rate of NE into the extravascular space, as well as other parameters to more fully understand the complexities of systemic and organ-specific sympathetic nervous system activity.

rates increased as LV end-systolic volume increased or EF declined. Thus, the systemic sympathetic nervous system would appear to accelerate or enhance its activity as the disease progresses. Although assessing the organ-specific cardiac specific sympathetic nervous system is much more difficult because of a complex input function, similar observations were made in that cardiac sympathetic nervous system activity increased as LV end-systolic volume increased or EF declined. This also suggested that the organ-specific cardiac sympathetic nervous system increases its activity as the MR process progresses.

Observations by Hochreiter et al. [8] have suggested that right ventricular (RV) performance is also of prognostic import in patients with MR. We have long known that MR is a biventricular disease because of its effect on pulmonary pressures and vascular resistance. Data support the notion that RV performance has an inverse relationship with pulmonary artery systolic pressure or vascular resistance, which may, therefore, explain secondarily the changes in RV size and performance. Because we had already documented that organ-specific cardiac sympathetic activity is related to LV end-systolic volume and EF, we tested the hypothesis that organ-specific cardiac sympathetic tone may also be related to RV performance and, therefore, provide an additional explanation for the changes in RV performance one observes in this disease process. Indeed, there was a significant inverse relationship between the activity of the cardiac sympathetic nervous system and RV performance, suggesting an additional mechanism for RV dysfunction in patients with MR.

β-Adrenergic Receptor Responsivity

Since systemic and organ-specific cardiac sympathetic activity is high, one would anticipate that the β-adrenergic receptor system is increasingly stimulated and may, therefore, be altered in its responsivity. However, identifying a direct relationship between indices of systemic and organ-specific cardiac sympathetic activity and responsivity of the β-adrenergic receptor system has been difficult, and a direct relationship between β-adrenergic receptor responsivity and contractility has not been established. Nevertheless, if the model for control of contractility is correct, the β-adrenergic receptor system must play an integral and important part in control of contractile performance. To test whether β-adrenergic receptor responsivity was related to contractility, we studied several patients with MR in the cardiac catheterization laboratory to measure elastance, an index of contractility [2], and obtained endomyocardial biopsies at the time of mitral valve repair. Our observations suggest that (1) the β-adrenergic receptor system is under intense stimulation, and (2) β-adrenergic receptor responsivity is related to in vivo contractility. We demonstrated a strong inverse relationship between basal cyclic AMP levels and elastance suggesting an intensely stimulated β-adrenergic receptor system. There were also strong positive relationships between the percent increase in cyclic AMP production at different stimulation levels of isoproterenol and sodium fluoride and elastance, while there was no relationship between the percent increase in cyclic AMP following forskolin administration and elastance. These data suggest impairments in the responsivity of the β-adrenergic receptor system at the β_1-adrenergic receptor and at the G-transduction protein, but no impairment in the ability of adenylyl cyclase to convert ATP to cyclic AMP.

Myocardial and Systemic Cytokines

Although it was clear that the systemic and organ-specific cardiac sympathetic nervous systems were activated and specifically related to LV size and functional parameters, there are other neurohumoral agents that the myocardium can produce which affect myocardial performance. One group, the cytokines, can be stimulated in the myocardium following stretch [9] or sympathetic activation [10]. Since one can surmise in MR that there is stretch on the myocytes produced by the LV volume overload and the organ-specific sympathetic nervous system is activated, it is not unreasonable to suggest that cytokine production in the myocardium may also be activated and, therefore, contribute to the myocardial dysfunction observed in this disease process. In addition, there are several mechanisms by which cytokines can alter myocyte function. These occur through inducible NO synthase, the neutral sphygomelinase pathway, and altered β-adrenergic receptor responsivity, which may be modulated by inducible NO. These processes have variable time courses for induction of myocyte dysfunction, but they are also reversible. Considering that myocardial dysfunction in patients with MR may also be gradually inducible and reversible in some patients, it is reasonable to consider the possibility that cytokines may contribute to this process.

To test this possibility, we studied control subjects and patients with MR both prior to and 1 year following mitral valve surgery. We demonstrated that TNF-α, its two receptors, and IL-6 and its receptor are increased in the plasma of MR patients prior to mitral valve surgery in comparison to controls, and there is a significant decrease towards normal in these cytokines and their receptors following successful mitral valve surgery. However, we found no relationship between systemic cytokine levels and LV size or performance. Despite the increase in plasma cytokines in patients with MR, this does not indicate that cytokines are being produced by myocytes. To further delineate this possibility, we obtained endomyocardial biopsies from normal donor hearts and patients with MR to test for mRNA levels of TNF-α, IL-1β, and IL-6 normalized to β-actin mRNA. We found a substantial increase in the mRNA levels of these cytokines in the MR patients compared to the normal donor hearts. Moreover, the ratio of myocardial TNF-α mRNA normalized to β-actin mRNA demonstrated a strong inverse relationship with LVEF, as did the IL-1β mRNA/β-actin mRNA ratio. Thus, these data suggest that stretch due to the volume overload or sympathetic activation probably stimulate cytokine production in the myocytes of patients with MR, and cytokines may contribute to alterations in LV ejection performance. Moreover, if these studies are correct and reversal of this process in patients following successful mitral valve surgery occurs, then the effects of cytokines on LV ejection performance may be reversible in part and contribute to the recovery of LV performance in some patients following mitral valve surgery.

Clinical Application

Although understanding the pathobiology of MR is important to our comprehension of the progression of the disease process, we have long sought an ideal time to refer patients for mitral valve surgery when surgery can effect an excellent long-term outcome, but not be premature. We might suggest that this is reflective of entering a window of opportunity that may remain open for a period of time and then close heralded by irreversible myocardial dysfunction or advanced symptoms. Accordingly, we hypothesized that echocardiographic indices of LV size or performance may be able to identify those patients with MR and a normal LVEF that were developing or had developed early contractile impairment and who might manifest a beneficial long-term functional outcome if mitral valve surgery were preformed at this time. Using receiver operator characteristic curves, we found that LV end-diastolic and end-systolic dimensions and fractional shortening all had discriminatory power for identifying MR patients with a normal LVEF who had contractile impairment [11]. The most discriminatory function was an LV end-systolic dimension of 40 mm, in that patients with an end-systolic dimension of <40 mm had normal contractility, while those patients with an end-systolic dimension that exceeded 40 mm had contractile impairment. Thus, LV end-systolic dimension of >40 mm appeared to be a highly discriminatory cut point for identifying MR patients who were early in their disease process with contractile impairment and, therefore, might be entering that window of opportunity when mitral valve surgery would be most beneficial.

When these patients were followed long term with echocardiographic studies at 3 and 12 months following mitral valve surgery, there were very distinct responses depending on whether or not patients had a LV end-systolic dimension of <40 or >40 mm [11]. In both groups, LV end-diastolic dimension declined with removal of the volume overload and were quite similar at 3 and 12 months following mitral valve surgery. In contrast, those who had LV end-systolic dimensions of <40 mm had no change in end-systolic dimension, while those who had higher LV end-systolic dimensions demonstrated a progressive decline in this measure, so that, at 12 months following mitral valve surgery, there was no significant difference in end-systolic dimensions between the two groups. As a consequence, while fractional shortening declined early following mitral valve surgery (but remained within normal limits) in those with LV end-systolic dimensions of <40 mm, subsequently it remained stable throughout the year following surgery. In contrast, in those who had larger end-systolic dimensions and contractile impairment, there was a short-term decline in fractional shortening well into the subnormal range which recovered at 12 months to within the normal range and to an extent that this value was statistically indistinguishable from that of patients who had smaller end-systolic dimensions prior to surgery. This suggests that those MR patients who begin to demonstrate enlargement in LV end-systolic dimension, particularly as it approaches or exceeds 40 mm, may be developing early contractile impairment. However, if mitral valve surgery is undertaken at this point, before further increase in end-systolic dimension, contractile impairment may be reversible, with long-term preservation of LV ejection performance and excellent outcomes.

Conclusions

The pathobiology of LV contractile dysfunction is becoming increasingly clear in patients with MR. Our data indicate that this pathobiology may be reversible in some, if mitral valve surgery is timely. Reversal of these processes may explain the recovery in LV ejection performance and contractility following successful mitral valve surgery. More specifically, emerging understanding of the basis of deterioration in contractility raises issues regarding prophylactic therapy in patients with MR. Modulation of the sympathetic nervous system with β-adrenergic receptor blocking agents may delay deterioration, although there are no data to support this contention at this time. Nevertheless, this line of therapeutic reasoning seems plausible and should be considered in these MR patients to preserve contractility and delay progression of the disease process and the resulting need for mitral valve surgery.

References

1 Starling MR, Kirsh MM, Montgomery DG, Gross MD: Impaired left ventricular contractile function in patients with long-term mitral regurgitation and normal ejection fraction. J Am Coll Cardiol 1993;22:239–250.
2 Suga H, Sagawa K, Shoukas AA: Load independence of the instantaneous pressure-volume ratio of the canine left ventricular and effects of epinephrine and heart rate on the ratio. Circ Res 1973; 32:314–322.
3 Nikano K, Sugawara M, Ishihara K, et al: Myocardial stiffness derived from end-systolic wall stress and logarithm of reciprocal of wall thickness: Contractility index independent of ventricular size. Circulation 1990;82:1352–1361.
4 Starling MR: Effects of valve surgery on left ventricular contractile function in patients with long-term mitral regurgitation. Circulation 1995;92:811–818.
5 Ross J, Miura T, Kambayashi M, Eising GP, Ryu KH: Adrenergic control of the force-frequency relation. Circulation 1995;92:2327–2332.
6 Mulieri LA, Lauvitt BJ, Martin BJ, Haeberle JR, Alpert NR: Myocardial force-frequency defect in mitral regurgitation reversed by forskolin. Circulation 1993;88:2700–2704.
7 Linares OA, Jacquez JA, Zech LA, et al: Norepinephrine metabolism in humans: Kinetic analysis and model. J Clin Invest 1987;80:1332–1341.
8 Hochreiter C, Niles N, Bevereux RB, Kligfield P, Borer JS: Mitral regurgitation: Relationship of noninvasive descriptors of right and left ventricular performance to clinical and hemodynamic findings and to prognosis in medically and surgically treated patients. Circulation 1986;73: 900–912.
9 Kapadia SR, Oral H, Lee J, Nakano M, Taffet GE, Mann DL: Hemodynamic regulation of tumor necrosis factor-α gene and protein expression in adult feline myocardium. Circ Res 1997;81: 187–195.

10 Murray DF, Prabhu SD, Chandrasekar B: Chronic β-adrenergic stimulation induces myocardial pro-inflammatory cytokine expression. Circulation 2000;101:2338–2341.
11 Flemming M, Oral H, Rothman ED, Briesmiester K, Petrusha J, Starling MR: Echocardiographic markers for mitral valve surgery to preserve left ventricular performance in mitral regurgitation. Am Heart J 2000;140:476–482.

Mark R. Starling, MD, V.A. Medical Center, The Division of Cardiology,
2215 Fuller Road, 111A, Ann Arbor, MI 48105-2303 (USA)

Borer JS, Isom OW (eds): Pathophysiology, Evaluation and Management of Valvular Heart Diseases.
Adv Cardiol. Basel, Karger, 2002, vol 39, pp 25–38

Aortic Valve Disease – Etiology and the Role of Vascular Pathology: Is the Face of the Disease Changing?

Valentin Fuster, Adam Rosenbluth

Department of Cardiology, Mount Sinai School of Medicine,
Mount Sinai Medical Center, New York, N.Y., USA

Evolving Etiologies of Valvular Heart Disease

The history of valvular heart disease has paralleled the evolution of man as infectious etiologies have gradually been replaced by those associated with the increase in longevity in industrialized countries. In the industrialized world the incidence of valvular heart disease remains high; however, rheumatic heart disease has been replaced by degenerative valve disease particularly aortic valvular stenosis in the elderly and mitral annular calcification (MAC) as the dominant causes (fig. 1) [1]. One surgical series over 5 years found a decrease in post-inflammatory valve disease from 30 to 18%, stable congenital bicuspid aortic valve stenosis from 37 to 33%, and an increase in degenerative valve disease from 30 to 46% [2]. Appreciating the contribution of atherogenic risk factors such as hypertension, hypercholesterolemia and cigarette smoking is critical to understanding the changing face of valve disease today. Coronary risk factors are intimately related to valvular heart disease, the proximal aorta and the aortic valve can be considered as a single entity, and changes in one are not exclusive of changes in the other. Other emerging etiologies of valvular disease include autoimmune disease, vasculitis, infection and drugs (fig. 1).

Degenerative Aortic Valve Disease

Understanding the role of traditional cardiovascular risk factors in valvular heart disease has derived in large part from observation of clinical factors

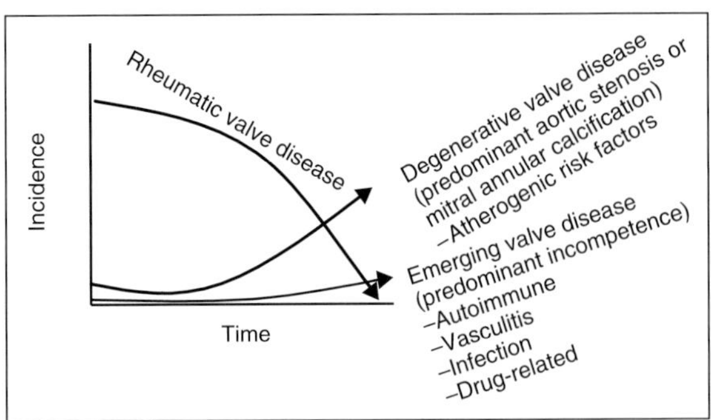

Fig. 1. Evolving etiologies of valvular disease in developed countries [from 1, with permission].

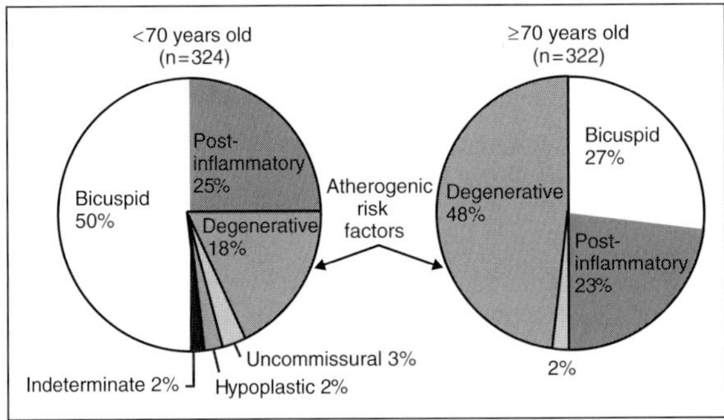

Fig. 2. Etiologies of aortic valve stenosis [from 2, with permission].

associated with the progression of degenerative aortic valve disease. According to Passik et al. [2] at the Mayo Clinic, prior to age 70 the etiologies of aortic valve stenosis include bicuspid aortic valve (50%), post-inflammatory (25%), and degenerative (18%). Above age 70, degenerative valve disease accounts for 48% and bicuspid aortic valve decreases to 23%, with post-inflammatory comprising the remainder (fig. 2). The increase in degenerative disease has focused interest on atherogenic risk factors known to predominate in this age group. A positive relationship has been demonstrated between age, male gender, smoking, hypertension, diabetes, LDL and HDL and the progression of aortic stenosis [3, 4]. Specifically, the Cardiovascular Health Study evaluated over 5,000 patients aged 65 years or more; aortic valve sclerosis was found in 26% and stenosis in 2% of the cohort [3]. Independent clinical factors associated with both pathologies included age (a twofold increased risk for each 10-year increase in age), male gender (twofold excess risk), history of hypertension (20% increased risk),

Table 1. Clinical factors associated with progression of aortic valve sclerosis and stenosis [from 3, with permission]

Variable	p value	Odds ratio
Age	<0.001	2.18
Male gender	<0.001	2.03
Lp(a)	<0.001	1.23
Height, cm	<0.001	0.84
Hypertension	0.002	1.23
Present smoking	0.006	1.35
LDLc, mg/dl	0.008	1.12

Table 2. Prevalence of coronary artery disease in older men and women with and without aortic cuspal calcium [from 8, with permission]

	Coronary artery disease	
	aortic cuspal calcium, %	no aortic cuspal calcium, %
Men (n = 752)	57	38*
Women (n = 1,663)	54	37*
Men and women	54	37*

* $p < 0.0001$.

high lipoprotein Lp(a), low density lipoprotein concentration; in addition, the lack of a statin was positively associated with increased progression of valvular disease (table 1) [4]. Such studies demonstrate the important relationship between the risk factors in the progression of degenerative valvular disease and atherogenesis in the coronary arteries, and have introduced the concept that by addressing the conventional risk factors for coronary artery disease, the progression of valvular disease may be delayed.

An intriguing positive relationship has been demonstrated between valvular calcification by echocardiogram and the prevalence of coronary artery disease (table 2). The early lesions of aortic calcification appear to involve an active process similar to atherosclerosis with lipid deposition (apo B, apo(a), and apo E), and macrophage infiltration [1]. Studies on surgically excised valves have demonstrated that the early stages of atherogenesis can also be seen in aortic valvular disease. For example, the same adhesion molecules (ICAM-1 and VCAM-1) which influence macrophages in the progression of atherogenesis have been found on diseased aortic valves [5]. The argument to be made from these studies is that degenerative valve disease is not simply a consequence of aging, but likely shares not only genetic similarities with atherogenesis, but also certain preventable or modifiable attributes. As such the same principles applied to decreasing the incidence of significant coronary artery disease, including dietary modification, tobacco cessation, plasma lipid monitoring and therapy, as well as blood pressure control could be applied to valvular heart disease.

Degenerative Mitral Valve Disease

The mitral valve is subject to the same degenerative processes as the aortic valve. The etiologies of mitral valve incompetence include chronic rheumatic disease, MAC, acute infective endocarditis, chronic myxomatous valve (MVP), acute flail leaflet, chronic dilated cardiomyopathy, and myocardial infarction. MAC is a chronic degenerative non-inflammatory process in the fibrous base of the mitral valve with increased incidence in the elderly and women [6]. Similar to degenerative aortic valve disease, studies have shown an association between MAC and atherosclerotic risk factors. Patients with MAC have a higher incidence of left atrial enlargement, hypertrophic cardiomyopathy, atrial fibrillation, cerebrovascular accidents, aortic valve calcification and aortic stenosis [6, 7]. Analysis of over 8,000 consecutive patients demonstrated age, hypertension, diabetes mellitus and hypercholesterolemia were highly correlated with both MAC and stenotic and non-stenotic aortic valve calcification. While calcification of the aortic valve with or without aortic stenosis may be a more serious process, the consequences of the same calcifications on the mitral valve, particularly the undersurface of the posterior leaflet, can be mitral insufficiency and rarely mitral stenosis.

Adler et al. [6] demonstrated a higher incidence of aortic atheroma, carotid artery disease, coronary artery disease (table 3) and peripheral vascular disease in patients with MAC. Pathologic studies on patients aged 13–39 years demonstrated foam cells on the endothelium of epicardial coronary arteries, ventricular surface of the posterior mitral leaflet, and on the aortic portion of the aortic valve cusps. At catheterization, among 165 patients with MAC compared with 147 controls without MAC, the incidence of stenotic lesions greater than 70% was 89% compared to 75% ($p = 0.001$); triple vessel disease 45% compared with 24% ($p = 0.001$), and left main disease greater than 50% was 13% compared with 5% ($p = 0.009$). In a population of more than 2,000 people with an average age of 70 years, a higher incidence of coronary artery disease has

Table 3. Prevalence of coronary artery disease in older men and women with and without MAC [from 8, with permission]

	Coronary artery disease	
	MAC, %	No MAC, %
Men (n = 752)	55*	40†
Women (n = 1,663)	51*	36†
Men and women	52	37†

*p = 0.0001, †p = 0.0001.

been found in those patients with MAC as compared with no MAC [8]. Such results are consistent with the increased frequency of cardiovascular events in patients with MAC.

Associated Pathologies of the Aorta and the Aortic Valve

As the etiology of valvular heart disease changes, associated pathology has evolved as well. Traditionally with aortic valve disease attention has focused on changes in the left ventricular size and function; however, older patients are now presenting with disease of the aortic root in association with aortic and/or mitral valve disease. Four disease processes demonstrate the integration of the aortic root and aortic valve incompetence: (1) chronic aneurysm of the ascending aorta, (2) acute aortic dissection, (3) chronic rheumatic valve disease, and (4) acute infective endocarditis (fig. 3, 4) [9].

Aside form its association with hypertension, chronic dilatation of the ascending aorta is commonly associated with a bicuspid aortic valve, particularly in patients with hypertension (fig. 5). Sabet et al. [10] at the Mayo Clinic have demonstrated that a bicuspid aortic valve leads mainly to aortic stenosis, but regurgitation, or a combination of both stenosis and regurgitation also occurs (fig. 6). At the present time a bicuspid aortic valve affects 1% of the population and 11% of first-degree relatives of those patients who have a bicuspid aortic valve (fig. 7) [11]. In patients with a bicuspid aortic valve, 58% have aortic root dilatation >34 mm compared with 20% of controls [12], and 9–18% of aortic dissections occur in patients with a bicuspid aortic valve [13]. The pathology that links a bicuspid aortic valve and aortic root dilatation may be found in a similar genetic origin leading to cystic medial necrosis with apoptosis of the media [14].

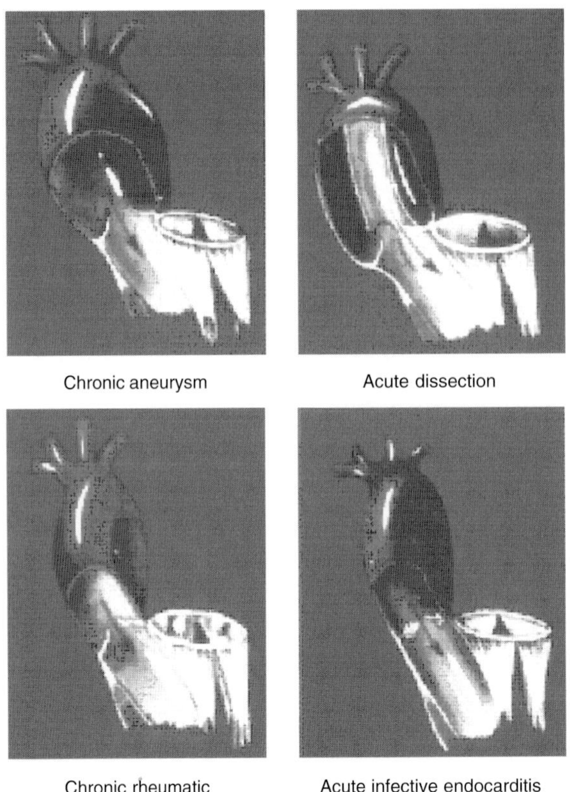

Fig. 3. Etiology of aortic valve incompetence.

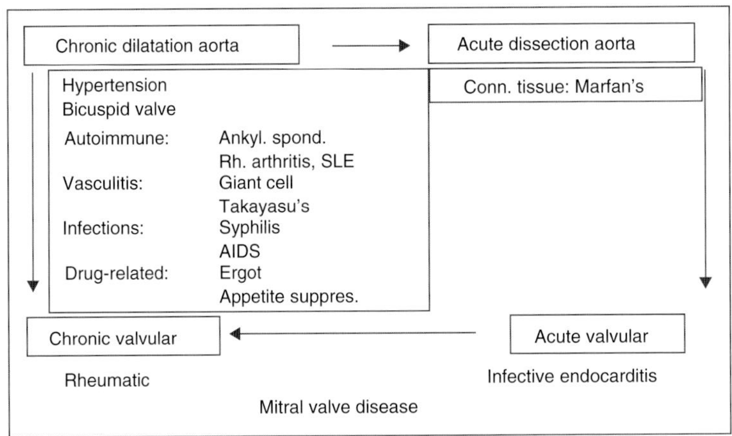

Fig. 4. Aortic valve disease (predominant incompetence).

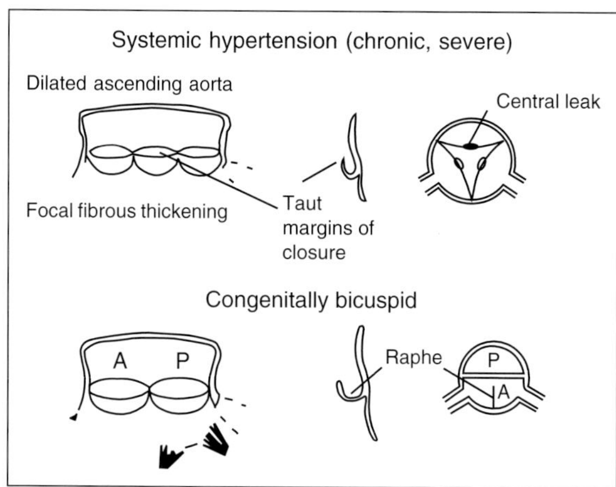

Fig. 5. Aortic valve disease and vascular pathology – systemic hypertension and congenitally bicuspid [reproduced with permission from Davis Co.].

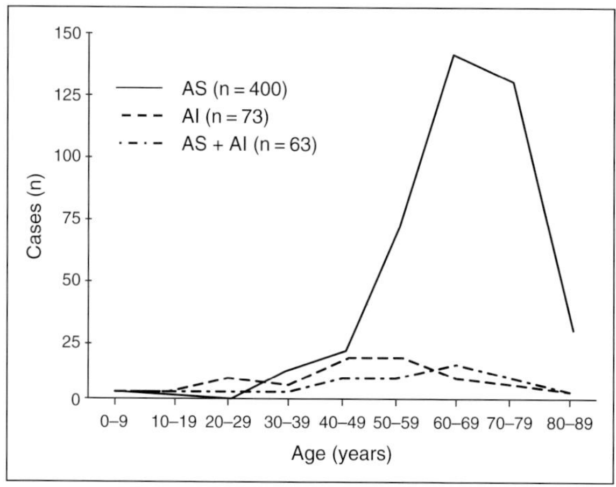

Fig. 6. Congenital bicuspid aortic valve (n = 535) age and functional state [from 10, with permission].

Although rare among etiologies of aortic stenosis, autoimmune diseases such as systemic lupus erythematosus, rheumatoid involvement, and ankylosing spondilytis (AS) demonstrate the role of inflammation in aortic valve and root disease (fig. 8). A high incidence of disease of the aortic root is found in patients suffering from AS, which is also associated with mitral valve disease. AS is an

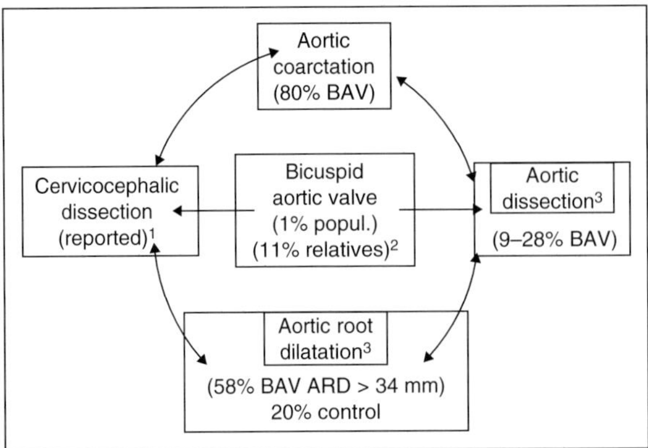

Fig. 7. Bicuspid aortic valve (BAV) – aortic wall. [3]Root Dil: Cardiology 1996;11:501; Keane et al.: Circulation 2000;102:III-35. [1]*Elastic locus:* Ewart et al.: Nat Genet 1993;3:11; [3]Necr and de Sa et al.: JTCS 1999;118:588. *Apoptosis media:* Bonderman et al.: Circulation 1999;29:2138. [2]*Familial:* Huntington et al.: JACC 1997;30:1809. [3]*Dissection:* Pachulski et al.: AJC 1991;67:781; Hahn et al.: JACC 1992;19:293 [reproduced with permission from Lippincott Wilkins & Williams].

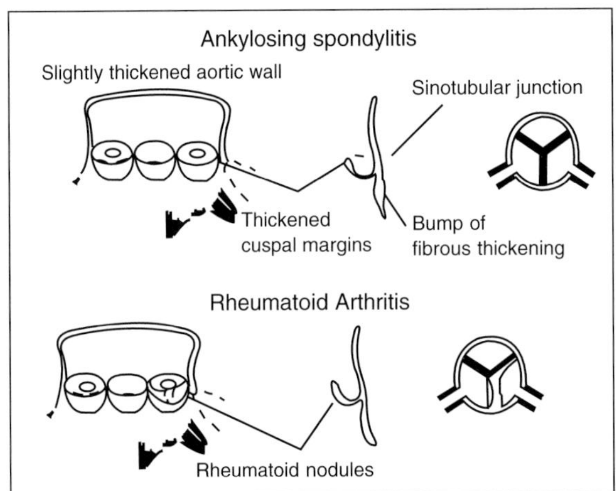

Fig. 8. Aortic valve disease and vascular pathology – ankylosing spondylitis and rheumatic arthritis [reproduced with permission from Davis Co.].

inflammatory process affecting the aortic root and aortic valve leading to aortic insufficiency. In a study of 44 patients with AS, 82% had an abnormality of the aortic root and/or aortic or mitral valve on TEE compared with 27% of controls (table 4) [15].

Table 4. Ankylosing spondylitis aortic root and valve abnormalities on transesophageal echocardiogram (TEE) [from 15, with permission]

Abnormality	Patients (n = 44)		Controls (n = 30)		p value
	n	%	n	%	
Aortic root abnormality					
Thickening	27	61	2	7	<0.001
Dilatation	11	25	2	7	0.06
Abnormal Ep or stiffness	27	61	3	10	<0.001
Valve abnormality					
Thickening	21	48	3	10	<0.001
Aortic	18	41	3	10	0.04
Mitral	15	34	1	3	<0.001
Regurgitation	20	45	1	3	<0.001
Aortic	7	16	0	0	0.02
Mitral	14	32	1	3	0.003
Tricuspid	1	2	0	0	
Any	36	82	8	27	<0.001

Ep = Peterson's pressure-strain elastic modulus.

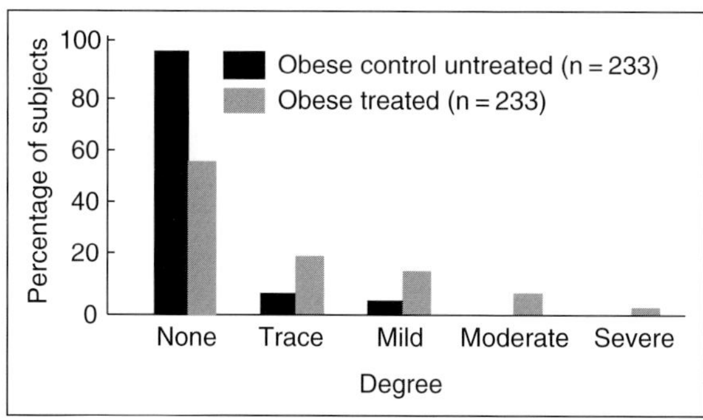

Fig. 9. Valvular insufficiency on echo Doppler in obese patients on appetite suppressants [from 19, with permission].

While studies of appetite-suppressant drugs and valvular disease have demonstrated a significantly higher incidence of aortic and or mitral valve incompetence among users of these medications, it is important to realize that in most of these patients the regurgitation is trace or mild (fig. 9) [16]. In addition, the magnitude

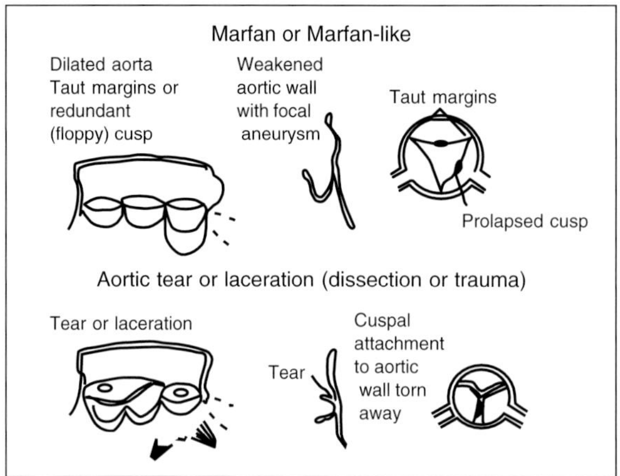

Fig. 10. Aortic valve disease and vascular pathology – Marfan or Marfan-like and aortic tear or laceration (dissection or trauma) [reproduced with permission from Davis Co.].

of echocardiographic valvular regurgitation varied between studies from 6.9 to 25%. Factors that may be involved in the differences include type of appetite-suppressant therapy, dosage and duration of therapy.

The pathophysiology is presumed secondary to increased serotonin levels in the blood contributing to a fibrotic process on the valve, similar to carcinoid syndrome [17]. The process can begin soon after initiating appetite-suppressant therapy, within the first 2–3 months [18]. Once the drugs are discontinued, the valve pathology may stabilize, and even improve [19]. As such, patients presenting with valvular incompetence on appetite-suppressant therapy who discontinue use should be observed for regression.

Acute Dissection of the Aorta and Marfan's Syndrome

In Marfan's syndrome, aortic valve insufficiency is a consequence of aortic root dilatation. A weakened aortic wall can lead to focal aneurysm with aortic root dilatation, producing taut aortic valve leaflets at the margins and prolapsing cusps at the center with resultant regurgitation (fig. 10). Over time the weakened aortic wall of Marfan's syndrome leads to 11% of all acute aortic dissections. Among patients with acute aortic dissection, 25% develop aortic regurgitation. Among this group, 60% present with type A dissections.

Three steps define the pathogenesis of aortic dissection (table 5). In the normal aorta, wall stress is uniform; however, patients with aortic dissections have developed inhomogeneous wall stress. The normal elastic lamina comprised

Table 5. Pathogenesis of aortic dissection from wall to hematoma tear to propagation [from 9, with permission]

Chronic pathophysiology of wall
Normal: Wall stress uniform – EL distributes
EL:30 sheets folded (media) – 5 fenestrated (vasa vasorum)
Abnormal: Wall stress inhomogeneity
Fibrosis – cystic (EL straight and replaced): hypertension – age
Fibrillin gene Cr 15/5 and cystic spaces (↓ quality): Marfan's familial (penetrance = degree mutation)
Dilatation: More wall stress (Laplace's law): hypertension

Acute hematoma and tear of entry
Hematoma: Rupture vasa vasorum through distorted EL
Tear: More wall stress and weakening

Acute or subacute propagation and tear of exit
Pulsatile flow: dp/dt and hypertension – valvular incompetence

of media and vasa vasorum is replaced by fibrosis, and worsened by hypertension and age. In patients with Marfan's syndrome, fibrillin 1 gene mutations on chromosomes 5 and 15 were recently discovered that lead to abnormal elastin, producing cystic necrosis in the vessel wall (table 6) [20]. The fibrillin gene encodes a large glycoprotein in the extracellular matrix, and this protein is widely distributed in elastic tissues. Marfan's syndrome has a high degree of clinical variability both between and within families. Each family appears to have a unique mutation in the fibrillin gene. Depending upon which mutation occurs there are a number of clinical syndromes that do not necessarily produce Marfan's syndrome, but may result in abnormal vessel wall elastic lamina. Rupture of vasa vasorum through distorted elastic lamina leads to the development of a mural hematoma. Increased wall stress and further weakening then lead to a tear in the vessel wall. What ensues is either acute or subacute propagation of the tear (table 5).

Mutations in collagen genes as a cause of connective-tissue diseases has helped to explain a history of aortic dilatation and dissection among families without any characteristics of Marfan's syndrome (table 7) [21]. Experiments were carried out to test the hypothesis that familial aortic aneurysms, either thoracic or abdominal, are caused by mutations in the gene for type III procollagen (COL3A1) similar to mutations in the same gene that have been shown to cause rupture of aorta and other disastrous consequences in the rare genetic disorder known as Ehlers-Danlos syndrome type IV [22]. A type III procollagen gene mutation produces an abnormal component of collagen in the wall of large vessels that caused synthesis of type III procollagen that had a decreased

Table 6. Marfan's syndrome: genetic disorders of elastic tissue

Fibrillin
Large glycoprotein component of elastin

Fibrillin gene mutation on chromosome 15[1–5]
Linked to Marfan's aortic disease
Linked to ectopia lentis
Linked to family trait (or sporadic)

Fibrillin gene mutation on chromosome 5[5]
Linked to aranodactyly

Variety of fibrillar gene mutations chromosomes 15 and 5[6]
Fragility relative to qualitative/quantitative fibrillin
Various clinical syndromes

Other fibrillin gene mutations linkages?[5,7,8]
Annulo aortic ectasia
Mitral valve prolapse

1 = Kainulainen et al.: NEJM 1990;323:935; 2 = Lee et al.; 3 = Masien et al.; 4 = Dietz et al.: Nature 1991;353:330, 334, 337; 5 = Int. Marfan Syndrome Collaborative Study, NEJM 1992;326:905; 6 = Milewicz et al.: JCI 1992; 89:79; 7 = Gibson et al.; 8 = Maddox et al.: J Biol Chem 1989;264:4590 [from Circulation 2000;102:IV-103, with permission].

Table 7. Genetic disorders of collagen tissue: non-Marfan's aortic aneurysms

Family history[1,2]
Frequent in aneurysms

Type III procollagen[3]
Glycoprotein component of collagen large vessels

Type III procollagen gene mutation[4]
Single family with aneurysms

Evolving prenatal – postnatal identification[5]
Automated rapid DNA testing

1 = Bengtsson et al.: Br J Surg 1984;76:589; 2 = Darling et al.: J Vasc Surg 1989;10:39; 3 = Prockop: NEJM 1992;326:540; 4 = Kontusaari et al.: JCI 1990;86:1465; 5 = Harrison et al.: Am J Hum Genet 1990;47:A219 [from Circulation 2000;102:IV-103, with permission].

temperature for thermal unfolding of the protein. Evolving pre- and post-natal automated rapid DNA testing is now available for these families. Such discoveries underline the importance of genetics and family history in dilatation of the aorta and problems with dissection.

Conclusion

The complexity of valvular heart disease is increasing and now requires an understanding of genetic diseases, congenital defects, acquired illnesses and known risk factors for atherosclerosis. Recent evidence has demonstrated similar risk factors – both modifiable and non-modifiable – for vascular and valvular pathology. As the incidence of degenerative valve disease grows with the aging population in the industrialized world, addressing modifiable risk factors is critical.

References

1 Soler-Soler J, Galve E: Worldwide prospective of valve disease. Heart 2000;83:721–725.
2 Passik CS, Ackermann DM, Pluth JR, et al: Temporal changes in the causes of aortic stenosis: A surgical pathologic study of 646 cases. Mayo Clin Proc 1987;62:119–123.
3 Stewart BF, Siscovick D, Lind BK, et al: Clinical factors associated with calcific aortic valve disease. Cardiovascular Health Study. J Am Coll Cardiol 1997;29:630–634.
4 Aronow WS, Goldman ME, Kronzon I: Association of coronary risk factors and use of statins with progression of mild valvular aortic stenosis in older persons. Am J Cardiol 2001;88:693–695.
5 Ghaisas NK, Foley JB, O'Briain DS, et al: Adhesion molecules in nonrheumatic aortic valve disease: Endothelial expression, serum levels and effects of valve replacement. J Am Coll Cardiol 2000;36:2257–2262.
6 Adler Y, Fink N, Spector D, et al: Mitral annulus calcification – A window to diffuse atherosclerosis of the vascular system. Atherosclerosis 2001;155:1–8.
7 Boon A, Cheriex E, Lodder J, et al: Cardiac valve calcification: Characteristics of patients with calcification of the mitral annulus or aortic valve. Heart 1997;78:472–474.
8 Aronow WS, Ahn C, Kronzon I: Association of mitral annular calcium and of aortic cuspal calcium with coronary artery disease in older patients. Am J Cardiol 1999;84:1084–1085.
9 Fuster V, Andrews P: Medical treatment of the aorta. I. Cardiol Clin 1999;17:697–715.
10 Sabet HY, Edwards WD, Tazelaar HD, et al: Congenitally bicuspid aortic valves: A surgical pathology study of 542 cases (1991 through 1996) and a literature review of 2,715 additional cases. Mayo Clin Proc 1999;74:14–26.
11 Braverman AC: Aortic dissection. Curr Opin Cardiol 1997;12:389–390.
12 Keane MG, Wiegers SE, Plappert T, et al: Bicuspid aortic valves are associated with aortic dilatation out of proportion to coexistent valvular lesions. Circulation 2000;102(suppl 3):35–39.
13 Pachulski RT, Weinberg AL, Chan KL, et al: Aortic aneurysm in patients with functionally normal or minimally stenotic bicuspid aortic valve. Am J Cardiol 1991;67:781–782.
14 Ewart AK, Morris CA, Atkinson D, et al: Hemizygosity at the elastin locus in a developmental disorder, Williams syndrome. Nat Genet 1993;5:11–16.
15 Roldan CA, Chavez J, Wiest PW, et al: Aortic root disease and valve disease associated with ankylosing spondylitis. J Am Coll Cardiol 1998;32:1397–1404.

16 Khan MA, Herzog CA, St Peter JV, et al: The prevalence of cardiac valvular insufficiency assessed by transthoracic echocardiography in obese patients treated with appetite-suppressant drugs. NEJM 1998;339:713–718.
17 Connolly HM, Crary JL, McGoon MD, et al: Valvular heart disease associated with fenfluramine-phentermine. N Engl J Med 1997;337:581–588.
18 Weissman NJ, Tighe JF, Gottdiener JS, et al for the Sustained-Release Dexfenfluramine Study Group: An assessment of heart-valve abnormalities in obese patients taking dexfenfluramine, sustained release dexfenfluramine, or placebo. N Engl J Med 1998;339:725–732.
19 Mast ST, Jollis JG, Ryan T, et al: The progression of fenfluramine-associated valvular heart disease assessed by echocardiography. Ann Intern Med 2001;134:261–266.
20 Tsipouras P, et al: Genetic linkage of the Marfan syndrome, ectopia lentis, and congenital contractural arachnodactyly to the fibrillin genes on chromosomes 15 and 5. The International Marfan Syndrome Collaborative Study. N Engl J Med 1992;326:905.
21 Prockop D: Seminars in medicine of the Beth Israel Hospital, Boston. Mutations in collagen genes as a cause of connective-tissue diseases. N Engl J Med 1992;326:540–546.
22 Kontusaari S, Tromp G, Prockop DJ, et al: A mutation in the gene for type III procollagen (COL3A1) in a family with aortic aneurysms. J Clin Invest 1990;86:1465–1473.

Valentin Fuster, MD, PhD, Department of Cardiology, One Gustave L. Levy Place,
Box 1030, New York, NY 10029-6574 (USA)
Tel. +1 212 2417911, Fax +1 212 4239488

Borer JS, Isom OW (eds): Pathophysiology, Evaluation and Management of Valvular Heart Diseases.
Adv Cardiol. Basel, Karger, 2002, vol 39, pp 39–48

Atrial Fibrillation and Valve Disease

John Somberg, Janos Molnar

Division of Clinical Pharmacology, Rush University, Rush-Presbyterian
Medical Center, Chicago, Ill., USA

Atrial fibrillation (AF) is the most common cardiac arrhythmia. While often thought to be a benign cardiac rhythm, we are learning that it is often associated with considerable morbidity, as well as mortality. The most recent Centers for Disease Control and Prevention (CDC) data reports AF prevalence of 2,000,000 and incidence of hospitalization of 353,000 per year. Patients with AF are at a considerable risk of embolization with associated morbidity and even mortality associated. AF with poor rate control can lead to important symptoms. However, adequate rate control at rest may often be lost on moderate activity or exercise. Poor rate control can lead to symptoms at normal activities of daily living, markedly reducing the patient's capacity to function. Additionally, the acute onset of AF needs to be evaluated looking for common causes such as poorly controlled hypertension, cardiac ischemia, hyperthyroidism or the possibility of occult valve disease. Indeed, as we will discuss, the acute onset of AF in patients with no valve disease may be a sign indicating worsening hemodynamics, that may necessitate an appropriate valve-directed intervention.

Epidemiology

AF is the most common cardiac arrhythmia and can be responsible for serious cardiac-related morbidity. The prevalence of AF doubles with each advancing decade of age, from 0.5% at age 50–59 years to almost 9% at age 80–90 years [1]. It is also becoming more prevalent, increasing in men, age 65–84 years from 3.2% in the period 1968–1979 to 9.1% in 1987–1989. The incidence of new onset of AF doubles with each decade of age independent of the increasing prevalence of known predisposing conditions. In the Framingham Study with a 38-year follow-up, men had a 1.5-fold greater risk of AF than women even after adjusting for age and for predisposing conditions. In the Framingham Study, hypertension and diabetes were significant independent risk factors predicting AF. Adjusting for other relevant conditions, heart failure was associated with a 4.5- to 5.9-fold excess risk and valvular heart disease a 1.8- to 3.4-fold risk of AF. In men, a myocardial infarction increased the risk for AF by 40%. Echocardiographic indicators of nonrheumatic AF included, left atrial enlargement (39% increase in risk per 5 mm increment), left ventricular fractional shortening (34% per 5% decrement) and left ventricular wall thickness (28% per 4-mm increment). Left ventricular hypertrophy (LVH) by EKG increased the risk for AF by 3- to 4-fold adjusting for age and 1.4-fold after adjusting for all other associated conditions. The Framingham Study found the primary adverse outcome for AF was stroke, which increased by 4- to 5-fold following AF. The risk for stroke associated with AF increased from 1.5% at age 50–59 to 24% at age 80–89 years. AF is associated with a doubling of mortality in both sexes, which is decreased to 1.5- to 1.9-fold after adjusting for other cardiovascular conditions. The authors of the Framingham Study concluded that AF is associated with a decreased survival across a wide range of ages.

New Considerations

Along with an awareness of the prevalence and severity of AF is an emerging understanding of a number of important aspects of AF. We are learning that prolonged excessive ventricular rates can lead to the development of cardiomyopathy in animals [2, 3]. Often, we have poor rate control with AF and thus this may be one reason that such a high association with congestive heart failure (CHF) is noted. Along with ventricular 'remodeling', evidence is developing that AF causes substantial changes at the molecular level; some of these changes are related to ion channel remodeling [4]. These changes facilitate further AF, making paroxysmal AF most likely to lead to persistent and then permanent AF. In fact, even short runs of AF shorten atrial refractoriness [5] making it more likely to have AF persist. Interestingly, the electrophysiologic changes observed with AF are somewhat reversible, more reversible the shorter the duration of AF [6]. All these remodeling changes have re-enforced the clinical observation that AF begets AF, an observation demonstrated in an experimental goat model of AF [7].

Outcomes with AF

The high incidence of stroke and other adverse outcomes with AF has been well documented by the Framingham Study. From the large randomized heart failure studies comes the observation that AF is associated with an increased risk for morbidity and heart failure progression in patients with asymptomatic, as well as symptomatic left ventricular systolic dysfunction [8]. These observations come from the SOLVD Trials that reported that AF patients compared to patients in normal sinus rhythm (NSR) had greater all cause mortality (34 vs. 23%, $p < 0.001$), death attributed to pump failure (16.7 vs. 9.4%, $p < 0.001$) and were more likely to reach the composite end point of death or hospitalization for heart failure (45 vs. 33%, $p < 0.001$).

Management of AF

When managing AF, a number of strategies are available to the physician. Acute management can be directed towards conversion or rate control. Rate control can be based on pharmacologic therapy or ablation therapy with the potential need for permanent cardiac pacing. While definitive data are not available to support conversion over rate control, most physicians will try to convert AF if it has not been present for a period of over 1 year, though often the duration of the AF is unknown or poorly known. Conversion can be accomplished through electroshock cardioversion or through pharmacologic therapy. Usually, conversion is also combined with pharmacologic pre-treatment to prevent AF recurrence in the post-conversion period. It is important to appropriately anticoagulate patients who have had prolonged AF, intermittent AF or AF onset of unknown duration. Only in those patients with a known onset of AF can elective cardioversion be undertaken. Emergency cardioversion is often done without anticoagulation and in this situation the risk of uncontrolled AF is balanced against the risk of embolization and possible stroke.

Acute pharmacologic therapy can best be considered in terms of the clinical problem being treated (table 1). A number of modalities to obtain rate control are available including the cardiac glycosides, β-blockers or the calcium channel blockers of the diltiazem or verapamil types. Intravenous amiodarone is also rather effective for rate control and has the added benefit of stabilizing the myocardium against ventricular arrhythmias, as well as converting AF and preventing AF recurrence. While digoxin prolongs refractoriness at the level of the AV node, it shortens refractoriness in the atrium, facilitating the persistence of AF [9].

Table 1. Acute AF pharmacologic management

Clinical problem	Goal	Therapies
Rapid rate	Rate control	Digoxin
		IV β-blockers
		IV verapamil
		IV diltiazem
		IV procainamide
		IV amiodarone
	Conversion	Ibutilide
New onset of CHF	Rate control	Digoxin
		IV diltiazem
		IV procainamide
		IV amiodarone
	Conversion	Ibutilide
Embolization	Anticoagulation	Heparin

Acute management can also include pharmacologically mediated conversion. Recently a new type III agent, ibutilide, has been approved for this purpose and found highly effective [10]. It exhibits a high degree of efficacy, but has the drawback of inducing a significant incidence of torsade de pointes ventricular tachycardia (VT) at times requiring repeat electroshock to terminate the torsade or ventricular fibrulator (VF) that has developed. Administering ibutilide to patients on amiodarone does not cause any more torsade and in fact, the incidence of conversion increases and the incidence of torsade appears to decrease.

AF and Surgery

AF following coronary artery bypass surgery (CABG) is the most common arrhythmia post-operatively and often is associated with prolonged intensive care unit (ICU) stay and hospitalization. Age, male gender, hypertension, intraoperative intra-aortic balloon counterpulsation, pneumonia and respirator-mediated ventilation for greater than 24 h are associated with a higher incidence of AF post-operatively [11]. In one study, the mean length of hospital stay after surgery was 15 + 28 days for patients with AF compared to 9 + 19 days for patients without AF ($p = 0.001$). The adjusted length of hospital stay attributable to AF was 4.9 days corresponding to over USD 10,000 in additional hospital expenses. However, these figures have generated some controversy and a more recent report has disputed these findings, reporting a 1- to 1.5-day increase in hospitalization [12]. These findings were obtained by adjusting the study for variables that may have independently prolonged hospitalization. However, it is our experience that AF does prolong hospitalization, though the current financial pressures often result in more rapid discharge than one would like, precluding evidence of the effect of AF in hospital day tabulations. AF is related to a considerable number of morbid events with a significant increase in re-admissions, peri-operative MI, CHF, stroke, re-intubation, 30-day mortality and 6-month mortality [13]. Additionally, the risk of AF increases from 28% with CABG to 30% with AVR, 32% with AVR and CABG, 41% with MVR to 55% with CABG and MVR [13].

Post-Operative AF Therapies

A number of therapies for AF post-operatively have been tried. Perhaps the most promising is the use of amiodarone. Amiodarone is available intravenously (IV) as well as orally, increasing its utility. The agent has minimal effects on contractility, is a mild coronary vasodilator and possesses β-blocking properties. While the drug long term is associated with protean serious adverse effects, the acute IV administration usually does not raise the concern of thyroid dysfunction, hepatic or nephrotoxicity or pulmonary fibrosis. Guarnieri et al. [14] have studied the use of IV amiodarone for the prevention of AF after open-heart surgery in the ARCH Trial (Amiodarone Results in Coronary Heart Trial). AF occurred in 67 of 142 patients (47%) studied on placebo versus 56 of 158 patients (35%) on amiodarone ($p = 0.01$). Length of hospital stay for the placebo group was 8.2 + 6.2 days and 7.6 + 5.9 days for the amiodarone group ($p = 0.34$). Morady and co-workers [15] evaluated 124 patients given oral amiodarone or placebo prior to cardiovascular surgery. Post-operative AF occurred in 16 of 64 patients (25%) in the amiodarone group and 32 of 60 patients (53%) in the placebo group ($p = 0.003$). Patients in the amiodarone group were hospitalized for significantly fewer days 6.5 + 7.9 ($p = 0.04$) than were patients on placebo. Total hospitalization costs were significantly less for the amiodarone group than for the placebo group (18,375 + 13,863 vs. 26,491 + 23,837, $p = 0.03$).

Sotalol is another class III agent that has been employed prophylactically to prevent post-operative AF. Morady [16] has reported sotalol to effectively reduce the incidence of post-operative AF. Gomes et al. [17] enlisted 85 patients in a multicentered study evaluating the effectiveness of sotalol. They found that between 80 and 120 mg of sotalol daily was associated it with a 67% decrease in post-operative AF in patients undergoing CABG. However, sotalol did not significantly shorten hospitalization due to an in-hospital loading period that needed to be added to the total hospitalization time.

Table 2. Chronic AF pharmacologic management

Clinical problem	Goal	Therapies
Rapid rate	Rate control	Digoxin β-Blockers Verapamil/diltiazem Sotalol Amiodarone
Arrhythmia persistence	Conversion/prophylaxis of recurrence	Amiodarone Sotalol Dofetilide
Embolization	Anticoagulation	Coumadin Low molecular heparin

Chronic AF Pharmacologic Management

The chronic management of AF can be approached according to the clinical goal envisioned. Long-term rate control can be obtained with pharmacologic management (table 2). Digoxin alone does not counteract the increments in AV node conduction seen with increased activity (sympathetic activation and parasympathetic withdrawal). Thus, digoxin therapy is often combined with a calcium channel blocker or a β-blocker. Both amiodarone and sotalol are effective for chronic rate control, combining a class III action with β-blockade. Both agents are useful in conversion and prevention of recurrence but neither shows the same very high conversion rate as seen with ibutilide. Low-dose amiodarone may be most effective and can avoid some of the toxicity associated with long-term amiodarone therapy used to prevent ventricular arrhythmias [18]. The results of the Canadian Trial of AF showed AF recurrence on amiodarone to be 35% versus 63% on conventional therapy (propafenone or sotalol). The selection of chronic therapy to prevent AF recurrence depends of many variables. The lower the patient's EF, the more likely to use amiodarone because of less pro-arrhythmia with this agent in patients with low EF. Sotalol is usually reserved for patients with a higher EF and those who can tolerate the stronger β-blocking properties of sotalol. Dofetilide needs to be adjusted for decreased glomerular filtration rate (GFR) and possible drug interactions. Dofetilide has been studied in a low EF population and not found harmful, but those patients with significant QT prolongation are subject to pro-arrhythmia and need to be excluded.

The use of flecainide and propafenone has also been studied. These agents are not safe in patients with CHF or low EF, and thus, their use in AF patients is problematic, except in those patients with normal EF.

AF and Valve Disease

In the context of valve disease, AF is common and potentially morbid. AF is often associated with mitral regurgitation. Pre-operative AF is an independent predictor of poor survival after mitral valve surgery for chronic mitral regurgitation [19]. As the atrium dilates, the atrial refractory period shortens and the vulnerability to AF increases, as demonstrated in isolated heart models [20]. In patients with mitral valve disease, left atrial dilatation predisposes to AF [21]. In a study of patients with left atrial dimension >45 mm, 68% had chronic AF, 4% paroxysmal AF and 28% were in NSR; when if the left atrial dimension was <45 mm, ⩾8% were in chronic AF, 25% paroxysmal AF, and 67% were in NSR [21]. Left atrial dimension also predicts post-operative cardiac rhythm. If the left atrial dimension was >45 mm, 66% of the patients were in chronic AF and the remainder in NSR while if the left atrial dimension was <45 mm only 5% of the patients were in AF and the rest (95%) in NSR after surgery.

The persistence of AF after mitral valve surgery can lead to thromboembolism and thus can nullify the advantage of mitral valve repair by requiring anticoagulation. The probability of serious rhythm disturbances resuming after mitral valve repair can be evaluated as a function of pre-operative rhythm [22]. Those patients with NSR prior to surgery had a 94% incidence of NSR post-operatively. Patients with pre-operative intermittent AF had a 79% incidence of NSR post-operatively. If the AF was less than 3 months in duration pre-operatively the incidence of NSR was 85% post-operatively. If the AF pre-operatively was 3 months to 1 year in duration the incidence of NSR post-operatively fell to 66%. If the AF pre-operative duration was 1–3 years then the post-operative incidence of NSR was only 35%. Furthermore, if the AF duration was 3 years or greater pre-operatively, post-operatively the percentage of patients in NSR was only 5%. Most interestingly, the authors of this study concluded that survival was similar in patients who had pre-operative NSR as compared to pre-operative AF. However, the survival differed in the patients who had post-operative NSR (92% survival) from patients with post-operative AF (77% survival) [22].

In another study, the most important prediction of survival following surgical correction of mitral regurgitation was EF [23]. Patients with lower EFs tend to have more AF and thus AF and low EF combine to designate patients with an increased risk for a poor outcome.

Although patients who develop AF usually show other symptoms or functional changes that would indicate the need for mitral valve repair or replacement, many clinicians would consider the onset of episodic or chronic AF to be an indication in and of itself for surgery [24–26]. In fact, Cooper and Gersh [27] have stated that 'the development of techniques for mitral valve repair has altered the treatment paradigm for severe mitral regurgitation. Surgical intervention before the onset of left ventricular dysfunction is recommended'. The authors include in their list of indications for surgical correction of mitral regurgitation the onset of paroxysmal AF.

In aortic regurgitation, Dujardin et al. [28] have preformed a multivariate analysis of predictors of survival and have found age ($p < 0.001$), functional class ($p < 0.001$), comorbidity index ($p = 0.033$), AF ($p = 0.002$) and left ventricular end-systolic diameter ($p = 0.025$) significant predictors. AF increased the adjusted hazard ratio by 4.53 ($p = 0.002$) for patients treated medically.

In the management of patients with new onset AF and mitral regurgitation or aortic regurgitation, the onset of AF should at the least initiate a new assessment of the patient. Have the ventricular volumes increased, left atrial enlargement progressed, left ventricular ejection fraction fallen? These questions need to be answered. The onset of AF should be treated as a significant new symptom raising the probability of the need for valve repair or replacement. The longer the patient remains in AF pre-operatively, the less likely it is to achieve NSR post-operatively. AF post-operatively will require anticoagulation and pharmacologic therapy for rate control, further complicating therapy.

Conclusions

AF is a common arrhythmia with serious consequences for increased mortality and morbidity rates. AF shortens atrial refractoriness, making persistence of AF more likely. Physicians have a number of therapeutic approaches to AF management. Ibutilide for pharmacologic conversion is available and amiodarone as well as sotalol have shown to be effective in preventing AF recurrence in a high percentage of patients. AF is common post-operatively and may prolong hospitalization. Pre-treatment strategies with amiodarone or sotalol may reduce the incidence of post-operative AF. In patients with mitral regurgitation or aortic regurgitation, new onset AF is a significant finding. Patients should be carefully evaluated with new onset AF. This finding may indicate myocardial deterioration, necessitating valve repair or replacement. Persistence of AF pre-operatively for greater than a year reduces the chances of post-operative NSR.

References

1 Kannel WB, Wolf PA, Benjamin EJ, Levy D: Prevalence, incidence, prognosis, and predisposing conditions for atrial fibrillation: Population-based estimates. Am J Cardiol 1998;82:2N–9N.

2 Shinbane JS, Wood MA, Jensen DN, Ellenbogen KA, et al: Tachycardia-induced cardiomyopathy: A review of animal models and clinical studies. J Am Coll Cardiol 1997;29:709–715.

3 Grogan M, Smith HC, Gersh BJ, Wood DL: Left ventricular dysfunction due to atrial fibrillation in patients initially believed to have idiopathic dilated cardiomyopathy. Am J Cardiol 1992;69: 1570–1573.
4 Brundel BJJM, Van Gelder IC, Henning RH, Tieleman RG, et al: Ion channel remodeling is related to intraoperative atrial effective refractory periods in patients with paroxysmal and persistent atrial fibrillation. Circulation 2001;103:684–690.
5 Daoud EG, Bogun F, Goyal R, Harvey M, Man KC, et al: Effect of atrial fibrillation on atrial refractoriness in humans. Circulation 1996;94:1600–1606.
6 Hobbs WJC, Fynn S, Todd DM, et al: Reversal of atrial electrical remodeling after cardioversion of persistent atrial fibrillation in humans. Circulation 2000;101:1145–1151.
7 Wijffels MCEF, Kirchhof CJHJ, Dorland R, Allessie MA: Atrial fibrillation begets atrial fibrillation a study in awake chronically instrumented goats. Circulation 1995;92:1954–1968.
8 Dries DL, Exner DV, Gersh BJ, et al: Atrial fibrillation is associated with an increased risk for mortality and heart failure progression in patients with asymptomatic and symptomatic left ventricular systolic dysfunction: A retrospective analysis of the SOLVD Trials. J Am Coll Cardiol 1998;32:695–703.
9 Sticherline C, Oral H, Horrocks J, et al: Effects of digoxin on acute, atrial fibrillation-induced changes in atrial refractoriness. Circulation 2000;102:2503–2508.
10 Glatter K, Yang Y, Chatterjee K, et al: Chemical cardioversion of atrial fibrillation or flutter with ibutilide in patients receiving amiodarone therapy. Circulation 2001;103:253–257.
11 Aranki SF, Shaw DP, Adams DH, et al: Predictors of atrial fibrillation after coronary artery surgery. Current trends and impacts on hospital resources. Circulation 1999;94:390–397.
12 Kim MH, Deeb GM, Morady F, et al: Effect of postoperative atrial fibrillation on length of stay after cardiac surgery. The Postoperative Atrial Fibrillation in Cardiac Surgery Study (PACS 2). Am J Cardiol 2001;87:881–885.
13 Almassi GH, Schowalter T, Nicolosi AC, et al: Atrial fibrillation after cardiac surgery. Ann Surg 1997;226:501–513.
14 Guarnieri T, Nolan S, Gottlieb SO, et al: Intravenous amiodarone for the prevention of atrial fibrillation after open heart surgery: The Amiodarone Reduction in Coronary Heart (ARCH) Trial. J Am Coll Cardiol 1999;34:343–347.
15 Daoud EG, Strickberger SA, Man KC, et al: Preoperative amiodarone as prophylaxis against atrial fibrillation after heart surgery. N Engl J Med 1997;337:1785–1791.
16 Morady F: Prevention of atrial fibrillation in the postoperative cardiac patient: Significance of oral class III antiarrhythmic agents. Am J Cardiol 1999;84:156R–160R.
17 Gomes JA, Ip J, Santoni-Rugiu F, et al: Oral *d,l*-sotalol reduces the incidence of postoperative atrial fibrillation in coronary artery bypass surgery patients: A randomized, double-blind, placebo-controlled study. J Am Coll Cardiol 1999;34:334–339.
18 Talajic RD, Dorian P, Connolly S: Amiodarone to prevent recurrence of atrial fibrillation. Canadian trial of atrial fibrillation investigators. N Engl J Med 2000;342:913–920.
19 Enriquez-Sarano M, Tajik AJ, Schaff HV, et al: Echocardiographic prediction of survival after surgical correction of organic mitral regurgitation. Circulation 1994;90:830–837.
20 Ravelli F, Allessie M: Effects of atrial dilatation on refractory period and vulnerability to atrial fibrillation in the isolated Langendorff-perfused rabbit heart. Circulation 1997;96: 1686–1695.
21 Sherrid MV, Clark RD, Cohn K: Echocardiographic analysis of left atrial size before and after operation in mitral valve disease. Am J Cardiol 1979;43:171–178.
22 Obadia JF, Farra ME, Bastien OH, et al: Outcome of atrial fibrillation after mitral valve repair. J Thorac Cardiovasc Surg 1997;114:179–185.
23 Enriquez-Sarano M, Tajik AJ, Schaff HV, et al: Echocardiographic prediction of survival after surgical correction of organic mitral regurgitation. Circulation 1994;90:830–837.
24 Chua YL, Schaff HV, Orszulak TA, et al: Outcome of mitral valve repair in patients with preoperative atrial fibrillation. J Thorac Cardiovasc Surg 1994;107:408–415.
25 Horskotte D, Schulte HD, Bircks W: The effect of chordal preservation on late outcome after mitral valve replacement: A randomized study. J Heart Valve Dis 1993;2:150–158.

26 Chua YL, Schaff HV, Orszulak TA: Outcome of mitral valve repair in patients with preoperative atrial fibrillation: Should the maze procedure be combined with mitral valvuloplasty? J Thorac Cardiovasc Surg 1994;107:408–415.
27 Cooper HA, Gersh BJ: Treatment of chronic mitral regurgitation. Am Heart J 1998;135:925–936.
28 Dujardin KS, Enriquez-Sarano, Schaff HV: Mortality and morbidity of aortic regurgitation in clinical practice. Circulation 1999;99:1851–1857.

J. Somberg, MD, Professor of Medicine and Pharmacology,
Rush University, 1653 W. Congress Parkway, 1589 Jelke,
Chicago, IL 60612-3833 (USA)

Borer JS, Isom OW (eds): Pathophysiology, Evaluation and Management of Valvular Heart Diseases.
Adv Cardiol. Basel, Karger, 2002, vol 39, pp 49–60

Selection of Patients with Aortic Stenosis for Operation: The Asymptomatic Patient and the Patient with Poor LV Function

Blase A. Carabello

Houston VA Medical Center, Houston, Tex., USA

For the most part, management of the patient with aortic stenosis (AS) is straightforward. When the patient with severe AS becomes symptomatic, he or she only has about 2 or 3 years to live unless the aortic valve is replaced. Thus, symptoms indicate the need for prompt valve replacement. However, this review addresses two difficult management issues: management of the asymptomatic patient with severe AS at one end of the spectrum, and, at the other end of the spectrum, that group of patients with far-advanced symptomatic disease. In discussing these aspects of AS, it must be noted that there is little evidence-based medicine by way of large trials in valvular heart disease to help guide management.

Management of Severe Asymptomatic AS

The natural history of AS is demonstrated in figure 1, which shows that the asymptomatic patient with AS has an excellent prognosis with nearly normal survivorship [1, 2]. However, once the classic symptoms of angina, syncope or dyspnea on exertion develop, prognosis dramatically worsens. Half the patients with angina will be dead in 5 years, half the people who develop syncope will be dead in 3 years, and half the people who develop the symptoms of congestive heart failure will be dead in 2 years, without aortic valve replacement. The data from figure 1 were obtained in the pre-echo era when the severity of AS was harder to diagnose clinically. In 1985, Kelly et al. [3] used echo-Doppler data to study patients with a transvalvular gradient of at least 50 mm Hg and demonstrated that even with proven severe disease, asymptomatic patients had a good prognosis (fig. 2).

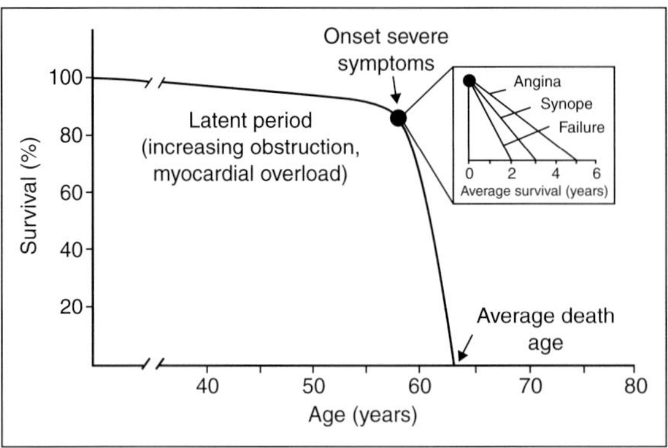

Fig. 1. The natural history of AS is demonstrated. There is a long latent period during which patients are asymptomatic and have nearly normal survival. However, once the classic symptoms of angina, syncope and heart failure develop, survival abruptly decreases [from 1, with permission].

Pellikka et al. [4] at the Mayo Clinic examined two groups of patients with Doppler-proven severe AS (fig. 3); 113 patients were referred for surgery because of symptoms while 30 patients were referred for surgery before symptoms developed. Outcome 4 years later was the same without any difference in survivorship between the two groups. In follow-up, Pellikka et al. [5] examined 610 patients with severe asymptomatic AS. The risk of sudden death in this group was 2%. Thus, all studies are in agreement: the risk of sudden death in asymptomatic patients with severe AS is small, about 2%.

The problem with waiting for symptoms to develop is that while asymptomatic AS has an excellent prognosis, the prognosis is not perfect. In each study a few patients who were monitored carefully experienced sudden death without symptoms or shortly after developing them [1–5]. On one hand, it seems unwise to operate on all asymptomatic patients since only 2% are at risk, a risk which must be weighed against surgical risk; on the other hand, medical therapy will result in a few sudden deaths. The obvious best approach is to identify a high-risk group upon which to focus. Otto et al. [6] (fig. 4) present data to help define this high-risk group. In patients with a peak transvalvular flow velocity of <3 m/s (peak gradient of 36 mm Hg), the chance of developing symptoms in the next 5 years was quite low, about 10 or 15%. On the other hand, patients who had a peak velocity of ≥4 m/s (peak gradient 64 mm Hg) had a 70% chance of developing symptoms and, therefore, required an aortic valve replacement in 2 years. Thus, the patient with a 4-m/s jet velocity is at high risk for developing symptoms.

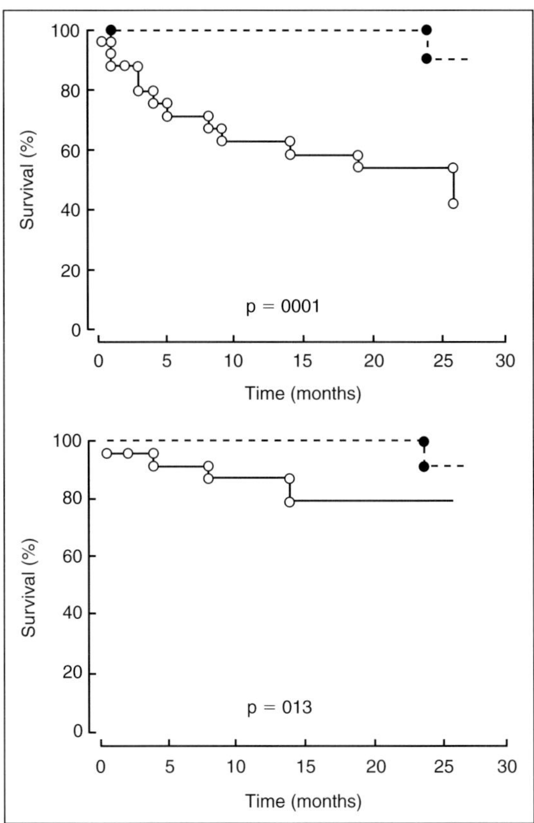

Fig. 2. All-cause mortality, cardiac death and sudden death are demonstrated for asymptomatic patients with AS (dotted lines) versus symptomatic patients (solid lines). Sudden death occurred in only 2 patients who had in fact developed symptoms 3 months prior to their deaths [from 3, with permission].

It should be noted that none of Otto's patients died, and all underwent frequent exercise testing. If those data are added to a recent study by Das et al. [7] which showed that exercise testing uncovers about 40% of patients who claim they were asymptomatic but 'developed' symptoms for the first time on the treadmill, they suggest that exercise testing could be used to further stratify this group of patients. While exercising symptomatic patients is most unwise, it appears from thousands of patients studied in Europe, that the asymptomatic patient can be exercised safely. In fact, patients exercise anyway since they are asymptomatic. Thus, it seems wise to observe at least one episode of physician-supervised exercise.

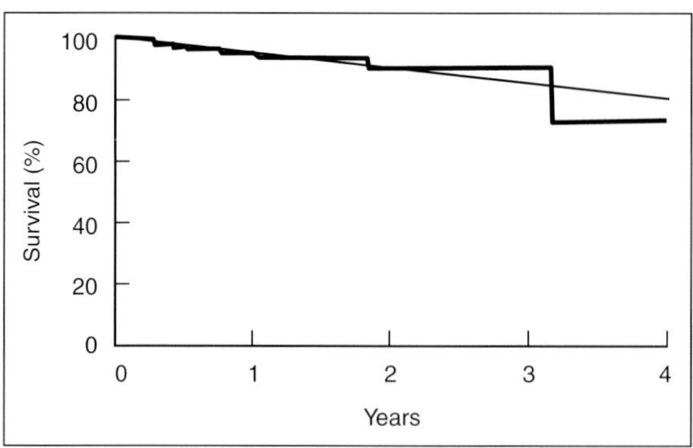

Fig. 3. Outcome for 113 patients with AS treated conservatively (thick line) versus 30 patients who underwent aortic valve replacement before symptoms developed (thin line) is demonstrated. There was no discernable difference [from 4, with permission].

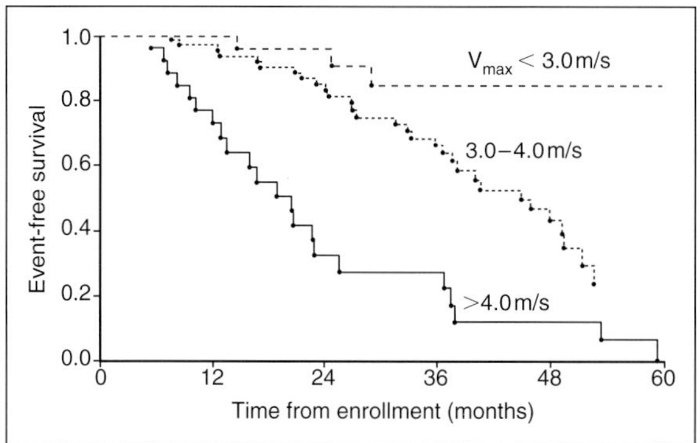

Fig. 4. Event-free survival according to transaortic jet velocity is demonstrated. Events were primarily the development of symptoms referable to AS. As can be seen, once patients developed a jet velocity of 4 m/s (peak gradient 64 mm Hg), the risk of developing symptoms was 70% within 2 years [from 6, with permission].

Therefore, the patient with the combination of a 4-m/s transvalvular flow velocity plus an exercise test that causes symptoms, hypotension or arrhythmia is likely to define a high-risk group of patients that may benefit from valve surgery even though they report no symptoms. In addition, patients should be instructed to report any of the classic symptoms immediately as opposed to waiting for their next office visit; aortic valve replacement should occur within the next 30 days after symptoms develop.

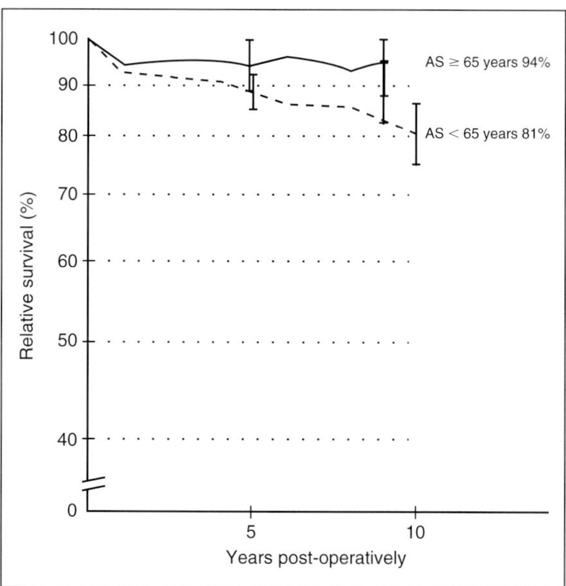

Fig. 5. Age-corrected survivorship is shown for patients 10 years following aortic valve replacement for AS. All patients did well and patients over the age of 65 had survivorship not significantly different from that of the normal population [from 8, with permission].

Once operated, prognosis is excellent (fig. 5) [8]. Age-corrected survival 10 years after valve replacement is similar to an age-matched control population over the age of 65.

Management of the Patient with Far-Advanced Disease

At the other end of the spectrum is that group of patients with advanced disease, pulmonary edema and low left ventricular (LV) ejection fraction (EF). For patients with low EF due to high afterload whose mean transvalvular gradient exceeds 30 mm Hg, prognosis is excellent because AVR reduces load and increases EF [9].

However, the most problematic patients are those with low gradient, low output and low EF. Carabello et al. [9] examined a small group of such patients with reduced EF (average 28%) and severe congestive heart failure (fig. 6). Transvalvular gradient separated those patients with substantial post-operative improvement from those who died or failed to improve. Outcome was poor when the mean systolic gradient was ≤30 mm Hg.

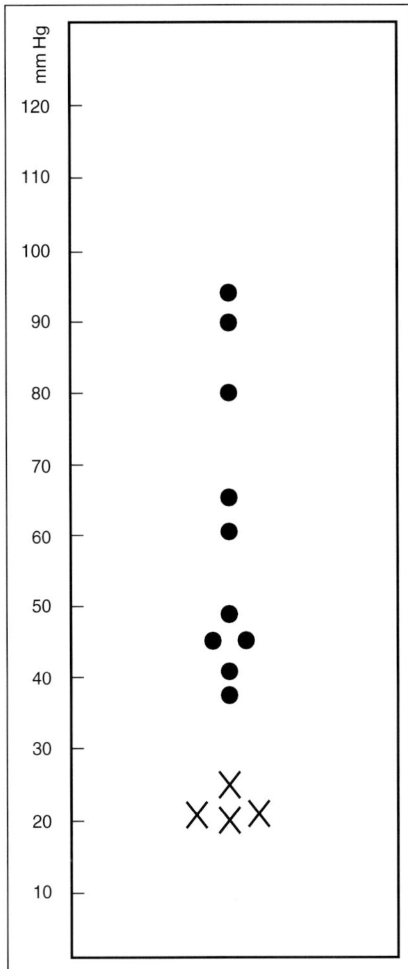

Fig. 6. Mean transvalvular gradient for patients with AS and low EF are demonstrated. Patients who survived surgery and improved symptomatically (●) had a much higher transvalvular gradient than those patients with the poor outcome (×) [from 9, with permission].

In a much larger group reported by Lund [10], post-operative survivorship was best in patients with a pre-operative gradient of 125 mm Hg and worst in patients with a low gradient (⩽35 mm Hg). Low gradient in such patients indicates inability of a severely damaged myocardium to generate force and pressure. Even the most recent data from the Mayo Clinic concerning patients with EF <30% and gradient <30 mm Hg demonstrated a 21% operative mortality; half the patients were dead in 4 years (fig. 7). However, while prognosis in this group of patients is poor, some patients do benefit from AVR. Following surgery in the Mayo Clinic study, EF only improved from 0.24 to 0.32 but the standard error was large; some patients had dramatic improvement in ejection

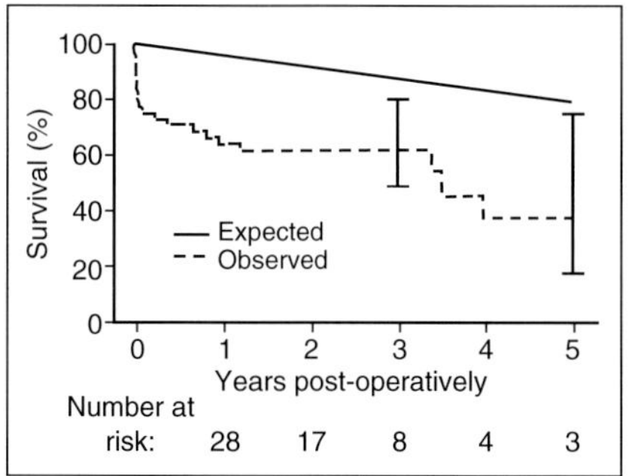

Fig. 7. Survivorship for patients with low gradient and low EF (dashed line) is compared with the normal population (solid line). The same group is compared to patients with a higher gradient As can be seen, there is a 21% operative mortality and only 50% of low gradient patients survive 4 years after surgery [from 11, with permission].

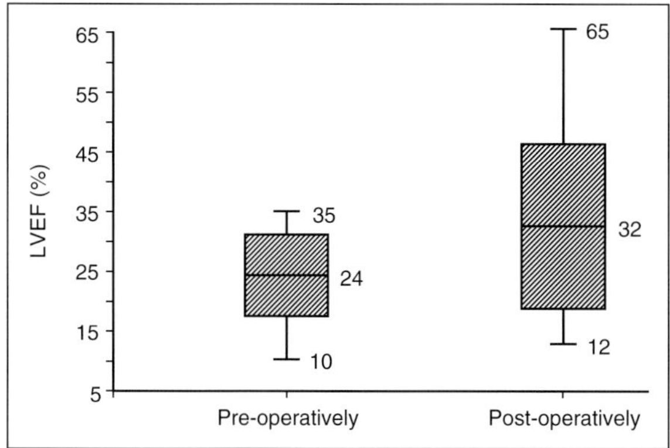

Fig. 8. Change in EF (pre-operatively) following surgery (post-operatively) is demonstrated for the patients shown in figure 7 [from 11, with permission].

performance following AVR (fig. 8). Brogan et al. [12] followed 18 similar patients: 6 died, 2 were unimproved, but 10 did improve. These studies point to the need to distinguish which low gradient low EF patients with AS will benefit from AVR versus those that will not.

The first goal in addressing this question is to divorce patients with true AS from a syndrome referred to as aortic pseudostenosis, a condition in which calculated valve area falsely indicates severe valvular obstruction. If severe AS has caused severe LV dysfunction, aortic valve replacement might lead to improvement because valve obstruction was the primary cause of the problem. However,

Table 1. Hemodynamics in a patient with AS

	Baseline	Nitropruside
LVP, mm Hg	130/30	125/20
AoP, mm Hg	100/70	95/60
grad, mm Hg	27	30
CO, l/min	3.0	4.750
PCW, mm Hg	25	18
HR, bpm	85	80
SEP, s	0.28	0.275
AVA, cm^2	0.5	0.9

AoP = Aortic pressure; AVA = aortic valve area; CO = cardiac output; grad = mean aortic valve gradient; HR = heart rate; LVP = left ventricular pressure; PCW = pulmonary capillary wedge pressure; SEP = systolic ejection period.

if severe LV dysfunction from another cause fails to open a sclerotic but not severely stenotic valve, valve replacement will be to no avail. The central problem in distinguishing these two conditions is that calculated valve area often cannot make this distinction.

Table 1 displays a patient with an initial cardiac output of 3 l/min, a mean gradient of 27 mm Hg, and a calculated valve area of 0.5 cm^2. At first inspection, there appeared to be severe AS. However, when cardiac output was increased by nitropruside infusion, the gradient hardly changed and calculated valve area increased dramatically. In this case, there presumably was a flexible, not severely stenotic valve, which a weakened ventricle could not open well. However, when afterload decreased and output rose, valve area increased.

Another way of looking at the problem is shown in figure 9. When resistance offered to outflow by the periphery (R_2) is greater than the resistance offered by a mildly stenotic valve (R_1), vasodilator therapy can increase output by decreasing R_2. In other words, R_2 is the major factor limiting obstruction to flow. On the other hand, if $R_1 > R_2$ (severe AS), vasodilators will decrease R_2 without permitting increased flow across the valve and blood pressure will fall.

To reiterate table 1, aortic valve area calculated either by the Gorlin formula or by the continuity equation is flow-dependent [13], especially at cardiac output of <4.5 l/min. As demonstrated in figure 10, if flow is increased through the valve, the calculated valve area will increase. This phenomenon has two explanations. First, the valve may actually open more due to increased flow. Second, the formula may be inaccurate. When Gorlin and Gorlin [14] derived their formula, they had

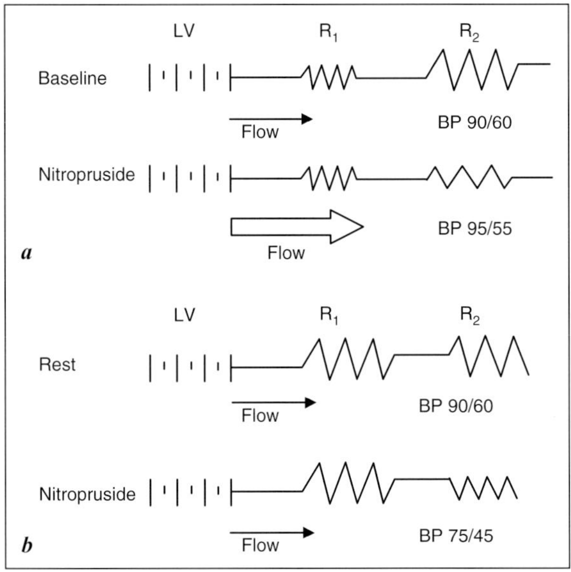

Fig. 9. ***a*** Aortic pseudostenosis, R_2 representing total peripheral resistance exceeds the resistance offered by a mildly stenotic aortic valve (R_1). When nitropruside is infused, both resistances become low and cardiac output increases substantially. ***b*** A true AS is depicted, at rest both R_1 and R_2 are large. However, following nitropruside infusion, R_2 decreases but R_1 does not resulting in no increase in outflow from the left ventricle but a fall in blood pressure (which is the product of cardiac output and total peripheral resistance).

no data for the aortic valve, and the discharge coefficients were therefore not calculated. Thus, some inaccuracy in this formula probably exists.

In severe AS, this increase in valve area with an increase in flow is small (0.1–0.2 cm^2). However, in aortic pseudostenosis, increased flow causes a large increase in valve area as shown in table 1 or, valve area becomes $\geqslant$1.0 cm [2, 15]. DeFillipe and Grayburn [16] demonstrated three groups of patients with AS and low flow to whom they administered dobutamine. In one group, valve area increased only by about 0.1 cm^2 when cardiac output was increased because gradient also increased proportionately. This group had severe AS and would be the group with the low gradient that might benefit from surgery. A second group had a large increase in output without a significant increase in gradient. These patients had mild AS (R_1 was small) and severe LV dysfunction. It can be predicted that these patients would not benefit from aortic valve replacement. A third group did not respond to dobutamine. These patients had no inotropic reserve. Recent studies indicate a poor prognosis for such patients [17].

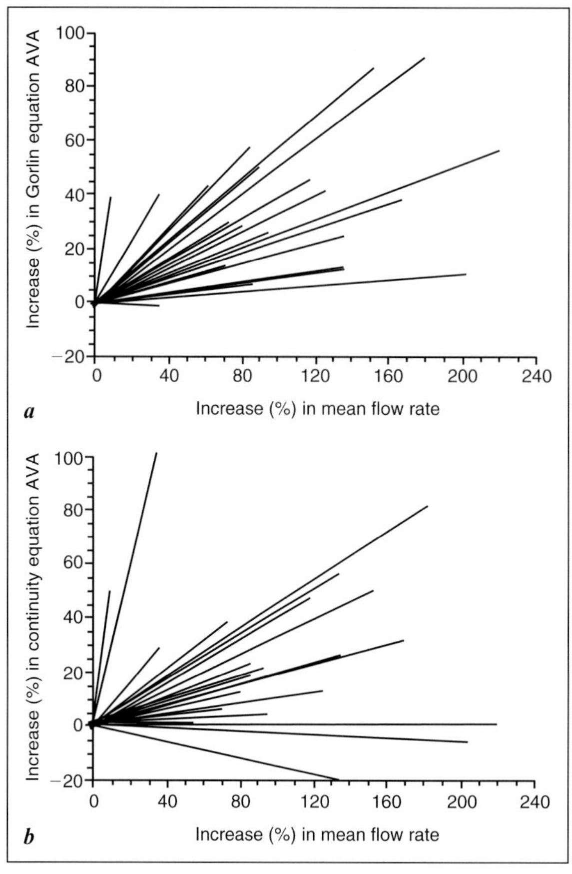

Fig. 10. The result of increasing mean aortic valve flow rate on calculated valve area by the Gorlin formula (***a***) or by the continuity equation (***b***) is demonstrated. In almost all cases when flow is increased, calculated area increases [from 13, with permission].

Conclusion

To conclude, asymptomatic patients with severe AS have an excellent prognosis, but a small group of such patients has a risk of sudden death. It is likely that exercise testing will reveal which asymptomatic patients are at risk by uncovering symptoms or hemodynamic instability. Exercising testing and close clinical follow-up, together with prompt surgery once symptoms develop, should further lower the risk of sudden death in this group. At the other end of the spectrum are those patients with far-advanced disease and reduced systolic ejection performance. Even in this group, patients with a mean transvalvular gradient

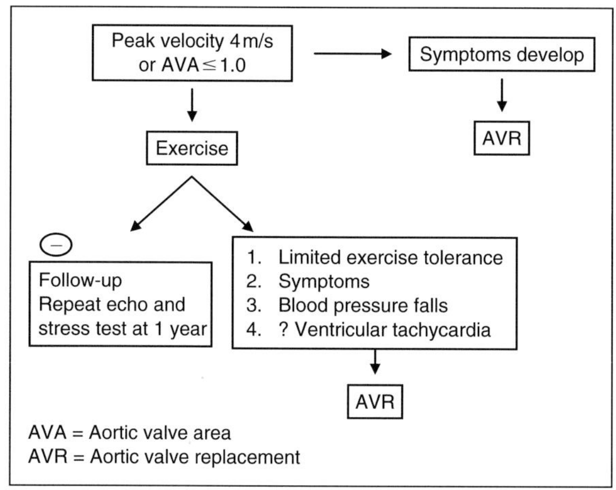

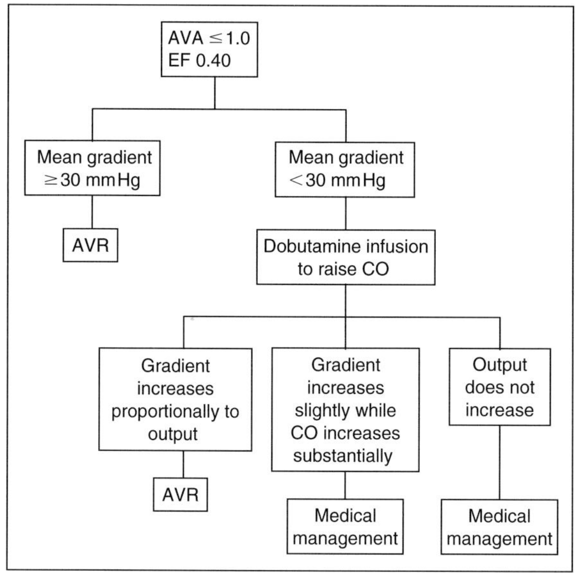

Fig. 11. ***a*** Management of severe asymptomatic AS. ***b*** Management of AS with EF < 0.04 and congestive heart failure.

of ≥30 mm Hg have an excellent response to aortic valve replacement. Most troubling are those patients with EF < 30% and mean gradient of <30 mm Hg. While prognosis in this group is poor, it is those patients whose gradient increases substantially with increased output who appear to have the best hope of improvement following aortic valve replacement. Figure 11 presents algorithms for managing these groups of patients.

References

1 Ross J Jr, Braunwald E: Aortic stenosis. Circulation 1968;38(suppl V):61–67.

2 Bonow RO, Carabello BA, deLeon AC, et al: ACC/AHA guidelines for the management of patients with valvular heart disease. A report of the ACC/AHA task force on practice guidelines (committee on management of patients with valvular heart disease). J Am Coll Cardiol 1998;32: 1486–1588.

3 Kelly TA, Rothbart RM, Cooper CM, et al: Comparison of outcome of asymptomatic to symptomatic patients older than 20 years of age with valvular aortic stenosis. Am J Cardiol 1988;61: 123–130.

4 Pellikka PA, Nishmura RA, Bailey KR, Tajik AJ: The natural history of adults with asymptomatic, hemodynamically significant aortic stenosis. J Am Coll Cardiol 1990;15:1012–1017.

5 Pellikka PA, Nishimura RA, Bailey KR, et al: Natural history of 610 adults with asymptomatic hemodynamically significant aortic stenosis over prolonged follow-up. J Am Coll Cardiol 2001; 37(suppl A):489A.

6 Otto CM, Burwash IG, Legget ME, et al: A prospective study of asymptomatic valvular aortic stenosis: Clinical, echocardiographic, and exercise predictors of outcome. Circulation 1997;95: 2262–2270.

7 Das P, Rimington H, McGrane K, Chambers J: The value of treadmill exercise testing in apparently asymptomatic aortic stenosis. J Am Coll Cardiol 2001;37(suppl A):489A.

8 Lindblom D, Lindblom U, Qvist J, Lundstrom H: Long-term relative survival rates after heart valve replacement. J Am Coll Cardiol 1990;15:566–273.

9 Carabello BA, Green LH, Grossman W, Cohn LH, Koster JK, Collins JJ Jr: Hemodynamic determinants of prognosis of aortic valve replacement in critical aortic stenosis and advanced congestive heart failure. Circulation 1980;62:42–48.

10 Lund O: Preoperative risk evaluation and stratification of long-term survival after valve replacement for aortic stenosis: Reasons for earlier operative intervention. Circulation 1990;82:124–139.

11 Connolly HM, Oh JK, Schaff HV, et al: Severe aortic stenosis with low transvalvular gradient and severe left ventricular dysfunction: Result of aortic valve replacement in 52 patients. Circulation 2000;101:1940–1946.

12 Brogan WC III, Grayburn PA, Lange RA, Hillis LD: Prognosis after valve replacement in patients with severe aortic stenosis and a low transvalvular pressure gradient. J Am Coll Cardiol 1993;21: 1657–1660.

13 Burwash IG, Thomas DD, Sadahiro M, et al: Dependence of Gorlin formula and continuity equation valve areas on transvalvular volume flow rate in valvular aortic stenosis. Circulation 1994;89: 827–835.

14 Gorlin R, Gorlin SG: Hydraulic formula for calculation of the area of the stenotic mitral valve, other cardiac valves, and central circulatory shunts. I. Am Heart J 1951;41:1.

15 Cannon JD, Zile MR, Crawford FA, Carabello BA: Aortic valve resistance as an adjunct to the Gorlin formula in assessing the severity of aortic stenosis in symptomatic patients. J Am Coll Cardiol 1992;20:1517–1523.

16 DeFilippi CR, Willett DL, Brickner ME, et al: Usefulness of dobutamine echocardiography in distinguishing severe from nonsevere valvular aortic stenosis in patients with depressed left ventricular function and low transvalvular gradients. Am J Cardiol 1995;75:191–194.

17 Monin JL, Monchi M, Gest V, Duval-Moulin AM, Dubois-Rande JL, Gueret P: Aortic stenosis with severe left ventricular dysfunction and low transvalvular pressure gradients. J Am Coll Cardiol 2001;37:2101–2107.

Blase A. Carabello, MD, 2002 Holcombe, Building 100, Room 4C211,
Houston, TX 77030-4211 (USA)
Tel. +1 713 7947070, Fax +1 713 7947377

Borer JS, Isom OW (eds): Pathophysiology, Evaluation and Management of Valvular Heart Diseases.
Adv Cardiol. Basel, Karger, 2002, vol 39, pp 61–69

The Value of Myocardial Perfusion Imaging for Diagnosing Coronary Artery Disease in Patients with Aortic Valve Stenosis

Andrew Van Tosh

Beth Israel Medical Center, The Division of Cardiology, New York, N.Y., USA

Angina pectoris is a common symptom in patients with aortic stenosis (AS), and may be caused by the AS itself, or by coexisting coronary artery disease (CAD). The goal of this article is to evaluate whether nuclear cardiology techniques, specifically myocardial perfusion imaging (MPI), can reliably identify the presence of CAD in AS patients. In particular, the review will focus on the question of whether MPI is sufficiently accurate that a negative study can exclude the diagnosis of CAD and obviate the need for coronary angiography in AS patients. The review will also consider (1) the prevalence of angina and CAD in patients with AS, and (2) the evidence underlining the importance of diagnosing CAD pre-operatively.

Prevalence of Angina and CAD in Patients with AS

Three-fourths to four-fifths of patients with AS have chest pain, and one-half to two-thirds of patients have typical angina. Paquay et al. [1] recorded an angina questionnaire in 76 patients undergoing catheterization for AS and correlated the results with coronary angiography. About two-thirds of patients with typical angina had significant CAD at catheterization, vs. 30% atypical chest pain; 5% of patients with no chest pain also had CAD. Mandal and Gray [2] determined the angina history in 73 symptomatic patients undergoing catheterization for AS. Angina class correlated directly with extent of CAD, and the severity of CAD correlated inversely with the aortic valve gradient. AS patients with more extensive CAD had lower aortic valve gradients, coming to attention earlier in the course of their AS because of their concomitant CAD.

A significant problem in inferring the presence of CAD in patients with AS is that angina may be caused by pathophysiologic processes other than coronary obstruction. One explanation for angina in patients with AS and no CAD is a mismatch between transmyocardial diastolic pressure gradient and flow necessary to support the increased left ventricular (LV) mass. There is also evidence that the coronary vasodilator flow reserve response is impaired in patients with AS. Marcus et al. [3] studied 14 patients with AS and normal coronaries undergoing valve replacement. They measured coronary flow reserve using an intra-operative ultrasonic flow probe and temporary occlusion of the left anterior descending coronary artery (LAD). They contrasted the patients to controls undergoing cardiac surgery for conditions not associated with LV hypertrophy (H). The patients with AS and (severe LVH) had significant coronary flow reserve abnormalities.

The recognition that many patients with angina have no CAD raised the question of whether these patients could be identified noninvasively, obviating the need for coronary angiography pre-operatively. Given the increasing sophistication of echocardiography for evaluating aortic valve hemodynamics, certain patients with a negative evaluation for CAD and well-defined AS by Doppler studies could avoid catheterization entirely.

Effect of CAD on Operative Morbidity and Long-Term Survival in Aortic Valve Disease

Whether coronary angiography should be performed in patients with AS is dependent on several considerations, not limited to the ability of scintigraphic techniques to rule out CAD. Other issues include whether CAD contributes significantly to peri-operative morbidity, and whether the presence of CAD affects long-term survival following valve replacement.

The contribution of CAD to peri-operative mortality in patients undergoing valve replacement for AS was reviewed in a meta-analysis by Georgeson et al. [4]. Four studies were reviewed, comprising over 700 patients. Aortic valve replacement (AVR) operative mortality in patients with isolated, pure aortic valve disease, without CAD, was 2.8%. In patients with CAD not undergoing coronary artery bypass grafting (CABG), operative mortality was 12.2% and in patients with CAD undergoing AVR + CABG, operative mortality was reduced to 6.1%. The presence of CAD thus has a significant effect on operative mortality.

CAD also has a significant effect on late post-operative mortality following AVR though the data for isolated AS are limited. However, in the Mayo Clinic series of 752 patients with predominant aortic regurgitation, the presence of CAD reduced 5-year survival from 82 to 68%, and 10-year survival from 63 to 39% [5]. In a study of 200 patients undergoing valve replacement for aortic and/or mitral regurgitation [6], there was excess long-term mortality in patients with CAD (22.4 vs. 7.4%).

Thus, for AS patients, peri-operative mortality and long-term outcomes following valve replacement are significantly affected by the presence of CAD. It is important to diagnose CAD pre-operatively since surgical treatment at the time of valve replacement may beneficially alter the natural history of the disease.

MPI for Diagnosis of CAD in AS

Factors Affecting Diagnostic Accuracy

There are several factors which affect the calculated accuracy of MPI in diagnosing CAD in AS patients. (1) In patients with AS, changes in loading conditions may have a significant effect on ventricular geometry, which in turn may cause scintigraphic perfusion defects. This was best illustrated by the work of Gewirtz et al. [7]. They demonstrated, in a canine model, that artificially created aortic outflow obstruction could produce scintigraphic perfusion defects, particularly of the apical region, which were indistinguishable from those caused by coronary stenosis, and thus could mimic CAD. Figure 1 is taken from this study. Control I is an anterior planar view perfusion scintigram produced by injection of labeled microspheres, and shows normal perfusion. In the same animal, experimentally created aortic outflow obstruction caused a moderate-severe anteroapical defect. Release of the outflow obstruction returned the perfusion pattern to normal in Control II. Temporary ligation of the left anterior descending artery ('Ligation') produced an anteroapical defect similar in distribution, but less intense, than that seen after aortic outflow tract obstruction. (2) The MPI technique employed may affect accuracy. Planar techniques are older, and in general are thought to be less accurate. (3) The definition of an abnormal scan also affects diagnostic accuracies. Early papers defined a positive result as any segmental defect, apical defect, or transient LV cavity dilation. Later studies included only focal defects as specific for CAD. (4) The stress testing modality used also may affect results. Early studies utilized exercise stress. However, the potential for hemodynamic instability with exercise in AS patients, and the realization that AS patients were often unable to exercise to 85% of the predicted heart rate, limiting sensitivity, led to the use of coronary vasodilator stress tests. (5) The angiographic definition of CAD is a determinant of the 'accuracy' of MPI. Studies vary between using a 50% versus a 70% luminal diameter reduction as the definition of hemodynamically significant CAD. (6) Pre-test likelihood

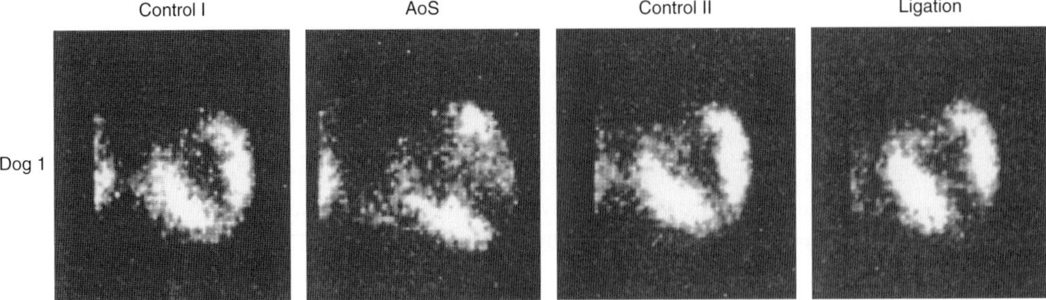

Fig. 1. Artificially created aortic outflow obstruction producing scintigraphic perfusion defects based on the canine model of Gewitz et al. [7].

of CAD clearly affects outcome in any single study. The accuracy and predictive value of a positive and negative MPI varies with the pre-test likelihood of disease in the tested population. Few studies catalogue the coronary risk factors or symptomatology of the cohort to gauge the pre-test likelihood of CAD.

Reported Diagnostic Accuracy

The studies using MPI to detect CAD in AS patients are shown in tables 1 and 2, grouped by the methodology of perfusion imaging: planar (table 1) versus tomographic (table 2). Details of the studies, including number of patients, criterion for diagnosis of CAD, percent of patients in the study with CAD, scintigraphic definition of an abnormal scan, stress modality and sensitivity, specificity, and positive and negative predictive values are presented.

The first study of MPI in patients with AS was performed by Bailey et al. [8] in 1976. They performed planar rest-exercise thallium studies on 22 patients, 11 of whom had CAD. A 70% lesion was taken as being hemodynamically significant. Focal thallium defects, as well as apical defects and transient LV cavity dilation, were considered abnormal. Using these three criteria, all 11 patients with CAD were identified, for a sensitivity of 100%. However, by those same cri-teria, 7/11 patients with normal coronaries also had abnormal scans. Consequently, the specificity and positive predictive value were low, at 36 and 61%, respectively. Figure 2 shows a patient from this study with normal coronary arteries at angiography. The rest image shows normal distribution of thallium. The stress image shows a severe anterior, apical and inferoapical (reversible) defect. The exercise image post-operatively was performed following an AVR only. Interestingly, all four 'normal scans' occurred in patients with no CAD, for a negative predictive value of 100%.

Four other studies have used planar thallium scintigraphy to evaluate a total of 68 AS patients [9–12]. Both exercise and dipyridamole stress were utilized.

Table 1. Planar myocardial perfusion imaging for the diagnosis of CAD in patients with aortic stenosis

Study	Year	Patients (n)	Dx CAD (%)	CAD (%)	Perf. defect	Stress	Sens. (%)	Spec. (%)	(+) PV (%)	(–) PV (%)
Bailey	1977	22	70	50	Focal, ap., diffuse	EX	100	36	61	100
Pfisterer	1982	13	50	41	Focal, ap., diffuse	EX	83	29	45	71
Huikuri	1982	16	50	44	Focal (ap. = nl)	EX	72	100	100	82
Huikuri	1987	27	50	44	Focal (ap. = nl)	DIPY	85	85	85	85
Roy	1998	12	50	33[1]	Focal	DIPY	100[1]	100[1]	100[1]	100[1]
Totals		90		44			87	64	66	86

[1] 4/12 had 'CAD' but 7/12 had CABG.

Table 2. SPECT myocardial perfusion imaging for the diagnosis of CAD in patients with aortic stenosis

Study	Year	Patients (n)	Dx CAD (%)	CAD (%)	Perf. defect	Stress	Sens. (%)	Spec. (%)	(+) PV (%)	(–) PV (%)
Clyne	1991	12	None	–	Focal	EX	9 (+), 1	cath = nl	3 (−)	No cath
Kupari	1992	44	50	48	Focal/ bull's eye	EX	90	70	73	89
Rask	1994	52	75	46	Circum. ct.	DIPY	69[1]	53[1]	–	–
Rask	1995	89	75	64	Circum. ct.	DIPY	100	75	94	100
							61	64	78	44
Samuel	1995	20	70	65	Focal	ADEN	92	71	85	86
Patsilak	1999	50	50	40	Focal	ADEN	85	77	70	88
Totals		267		46			86	72	81	82

[1] Calculated by vessel.

The definition of an abnormal scan varied as listed in table 1. The total sensitivity for all studies was 87%, specificity was 64%, positive predictive value was 66%, and negative predictive value was 86%. Thus, 14% of normal scans occurred in patients with significant CAD. A contributing factor to the limited negative predictive value may have been the fact that apical defects were considered normal in some series. However, 2 patients in the Pfisterer et al. [9]

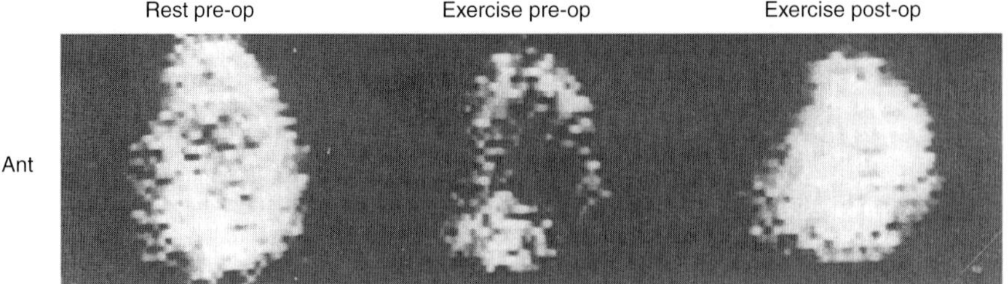

Fig. 2. A patient showing normal coronary arteries at angiography.

study had CAD despite negative scans, 1 with an 80% circumflex stenosis, and 1 with three-vessel CAD. One patient in the Huikari et al. [10] study had a negative scan despite a 75% stenosis of the left main coronary artery. The study of Roy et al. [12] reports 100% accuracy for dipyridamole thallium scintigraphy in 12 AS patients, 4 with CAD and 8 with normal coronaries. However, 3 of the patients they identified 'correctly' as having negative scans and no coronary disease underwent CABG along with AVR – casting some doubt as to the grading of angiography and estimates of thallium diagnostic accuracy.

Table 2 lists the six studies which used tomographic (SPECT) MPI to study AS patients [13–18]. A total of 267 patients have been evaluated. Included among these is the study of Clyne et al. [13], who performed exercise SPECT thallium MPI on 12 AS patients, only 1 of whom had catheterization (abnormal thallium scan but normal angiography). Four of the five other studies used pharmacologic rather than exercise stress. Only one study, that of Samuel et al. [17], used technetium-based tracers. Excluding the study of Clyne et al. [13], the overall sensitivity was 86%, specificity was 72%, positive predictive value was 81% and negative predictive value was 82%. The sensitivity and negative predictive values are comparable to those seen with planar imaging, but the specificity and positive predictive value are somewhat higher.

Figure 3 shows a SPECT thallium study performed in a patient with AS and angina at Beth Israel Medical Center, New York. The stress vertical long axis and short axis exercise images are pictured. There is a normal distribution of thallium tracer. At angiography, the patient was found to have a 70% lesion of the mid-portion of the LAD, and moderate AS. He underwent LAD angioplasty and became asymptomatic. Thus, figure 3 represents an illustrative case in which MPI failed to detect hemodynamically significant CAD in a patient with AS.

The first relatively large SPECT study of patients with AS was carried out by Kupari et al. [14] in 1992, in Helsinki. They studied 44 patients, 21 with CAD, using exercise-redistribution SPECT thallium, with quantitative bull's-eye map analysis. They distinguished between focal segmental defects, which they believe

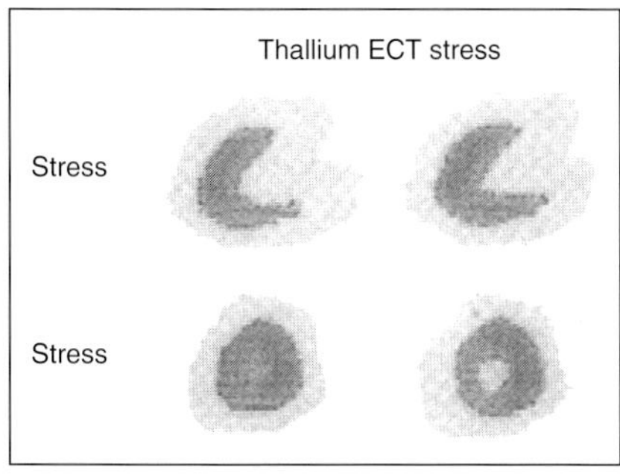

Fig. 3. An illustrative case in which MPI failed to detect hemodynamically significant CAD in a patient with AS.

were likely to be due to CAD, and diffusely patchy uptake, which they considered to be 'normal', and unlikely to be due to CAD. Focal defects were present in 19/21 patients, for a sensitivity of 90%, but were also present in 7/23 patients with no CAD. Echocardiographic studies were performed in all patients and showed that the presence of an abnormal scan in the presence of normal coronaries is associated with a higher gradient and greater degrees of LVH and LV mass. Interestingly, 2 of 3 patients classified as being unlikely to have CAD by thallium scintigraphy actually had >80% stenoses of their LAD.

The 1995 study by Rask et al. [16] used dipyridamole thallium scintigraphy to evaluate 89 patients with AS. The first 20 patients without CAD, MI, or LBBB were used to construct a 'normal file' bull's-eye database. An abnormal study was then considered one with segmental thallium uptake values 2.5 SD below the normal uptake levels on the bull's-eye map. Criterion for significant CAD was >75% luminal diameter reduction; 13 patients with >50% but <75% lesions were excluded from analysis. This is the only study in which data are presented by gender. Table 2 shows the accuracy for males on the upper row and for females on the lower row. Accuracy values for males were comparable to other studies. However, female patients had relatively lower sensitivity, specificity and predictive value. This may be related to the difficulty in distinguishing between anterior perfusion defects and attenuation artifacts in women.

The study of Samuel et al. [17] is the only series in which adenosine dual isotope studies (rest thallium, stress sestamibi) were performed. Twenty patients were evaluated. They were able to successfully identify 12/13 patients with CAD, but 2/7 patients with normal coronaries also had abnormal MPI. Six patients had normal SPECT studies, 1 of whom had CAD, the extent of which was not further discussed. Sensitivity, specificity, positive and negative predictive values were comparable to other studies.

The most recent study was that of Patsilinakos et al. [18], who studied 50 patients with AS using adenosine SPECT thallium, with rest re-injection performed for fixed defects. As in previous studies, they found a sensitivity of 85%, and a slightly lower specificity and positive predictive value. Three of 26 patients with normal perfusion had CAD – a normal scan in their series did not rule out coronary stenosis.

Conclusion and Summary

Angina is a common symptom in patients with AS with or without accompanying CAD. When due to the valvular obstruction alone, the pathophysiology involves mismatch between reduced diastolic coronary flow and increased LV mass, or impaired coronary vasodilator reserve. When CAD is present, the severity of angina correlates with the extent of CAD, which tends to be inversely related to the degree of valvular obstruction at presentation. It is important to make a correct diagnosis of CAD in AS patients pre-operatively, since this factor significantly influences peri-operative morbidity and long-term survival.

Whether MPI in AS patients can completely exclude CAD and eliminate the need for coronary angiography is a difficult question. Approximately 350 AS patients having had MPI have been reported. The studies differ in terms of scintigraphic technique (planar versus SPECT), stress modality, isotopes used, and definitions of an abnormal scan and what constitutes hemodynamically significant coronary stenosis. The 'best case' diagnostic data showed sensitivity of 87%, specificity 72%, positive predictive value of 81%, and negative predictive value of 86%. These figures indicate a high degree of accuracy and are comparable to the results of MPI in patients without AS. However, the data suggest that the diagnosis of coronary disease is missed by MPI in 14% of AS patients with CAD. Review of the referenced series indicates that in many cases, the stenoses were hemodynamically significant, and were important to identify preoperatively to avoid operative morbidity and improve long-term prognosis. Thus, in conclusion, although MPI is highly accurate in AS patients, a normal study cannot totally exclude the diagnosis of CAD. Coronary angiography should continue to be performed, particularly in patients with angina, or who are at risk for CAD because of their risk factor profile.

References

1 Paquay PA, Anderson GM, Diefenthal H, Nordstrom L, Richman HG, Gobel FL: Chest pain as a predictor of coronary disease in patients with obstructive aortic valve disease. Am J Cardiol 1976;38:863–869.

2 Mandai AD, Gray TR: Significance of angina pectoris in aortic valve stenosis. Br Heart J 1976;38:811–855.

3 Marcus ML, Doty DD, Hiratzka LF, Wright CD, Eastham CL: Decreased coronary reserve – A mechanism for angina pectoris in patients with aortic stenosis and normal coronary arteries. N Engl J Med 1982;307:1362–1367.

4 Georgeson S, Meyer KD, Pauker SG: Decision analysis in clinical cardiology: When is coronary angiography required in aortic stenosis? J Am Coll Cardiol 1990;15:751–762.
5 Tribouilloy CM, Enriquez-Sarano M, Schaff HV, Orszulak TA, Fett SA, Bailey KR, Tajik AJ, Frye RL: Excess mortality due to coronary artery disease after valve surgery. Circulation 1998;98:II-108–II-115.
6 Borer JS, Supino P, Hochreiter CA, Herrold E, Devereux R, Roman M, Kligfield P, Krieger K, Isom O, Yin A: Impact of coronary disease on survival after valve replacement for non-ischemic valve disease; in Lewis B, Halon D, Flugelman M, Touboul P (eds): Coronary Artery Disease: Prevention to Intervention. Proc Third International Congress on Coronary Artery Disease. Bologna, Monduzzi, 2000, pp 173–178.
7 Gewirtz H, Grotte GJ, Strauss HW, O'Keefe DD, Akins CCW, Daggett WM, Pohost GM: The influence of left ventricular volume and wall motion on myocardial images. Circulation 1979;59:1172–1177.
8 Bailey IK, Come PC, Kelly DT, Burow RD, Griffith LSC, Strauss HW, Pitt B: Thallium-201 myocardial perfusion imaging in aortic valve stenosis. Am J Cardiol 1977;40:889–899.
9 Pfisterer M, Muller-Brad J, Brundler H, Cueni T: Prevalence and significance of reversible radionuclide ischemic perfusion defects in symptomatic aortic valve disease patients with or without concomitant coronary disease. Am Heart J 1982;103:92–96.
10 Huikuri HV, Korhonen UR, Heikkila J, Takkunen JT: Detection of coronary artery disease by thallium scintigraphy in patients with valvular heart disease. Br Heart J 1986;56:146–151.
11 Huikuri HV, Korhonen UR, lkaheimo MJ, Heikkila J, Takkunen JT: Detection of coronary artery disease by thallium imaging using a combined intravenous dipyridamole and isometric handgrip test in patients with aortic valve stenosis. Am J Cardiol 1987;59:336–340.
12 Roy S, Hawkins T, Bourke JP: The safety of dipyridamole thallium imaging in patients with critical aortic valve stenosis and angina. Nucl Med Commun 1998;19:784–794.
13 Clyne CA, Arighi JA, Maron BJ, Dilsizian V, Bonow RO, Cannon RO: Systemic and left ventricular responses to exercise stress in asymptomatic patients with valvular aortic stenosis. Am J Cardiol 1991;68:149–176.
14 Kupari M, Virtanen KS, Turto H, Viitasalo M, Manttari M, Lindroos M, Koskela E, Leinonen H, Pohjola-Sintonen S, Heikkila J: Exclusion of coronary artery disease by exercise thallium-201 tomography in patients with aortic valve stenosis. Am J Cardiol 1992;70:635–640.
15 Rask LP, Karp K, Edlund B, Eriksson P, Mooe T, Wiklund U: Computer-assisted evaluation of dipyridamole thallium-201 SPECT in patients with aortic stenosis. J Nucl Med 1994;35:983–988.
16 Rask LP, Karp KH, Eriksson NP, Mooe T: Dipyridamole thallium-201 single-photon emission tomography in aortic stenosis: Gender differences. Eur J Nucl Med 1995;22:1155–1162.
17 Samuels B, Kiat H, Friedman JD, Berman DS: Adenosine pharmacologic stress myocardial perfusion tomographic imaging in patients with significant aortic stenosis. J Am Coll Cardiol 1995;25:99–106.
18 Patsilinakos SP, Kranidis AI, Antonelis IP, Filippatos G, Houssianakou IK, Zamanis NI, Sioras E, Tsiotika T, Kardaras F, Anthopoulos LP: Detection of coronary artery disease in patients with severe aortic stenosis with noninvasive methods. Angiology 1999;50:309–317.

Andrew Van Tosh, MD, Beth Israel Medical Center, The Division of Cardiology,
New York, NY 10003 (USA)

Borer JS, Isom OW (eds): Pathophysiology, Evaluation and Management of Valvular Heart Diseases.
Adv Cardiol. Basel, Karger, 2002, vol 39, pp 70–73

Congenital Aortic Stenosis: Is Repair an Option?

John J. Lamberti

Department of Cardiothoracic Surgery and The Howard Gilman Institute for Valvular Heart Diseases, Weill Medical College of Cornell University, New York-Presbyterian Hospital-New York Weill Cornell Medical Center, New York, N.Y., USA

Symptomatic congenital aortic stenosis (AS) may affect newborns as well as the elderly. The age of the patient and the pathological findings generally dictate the management. Isolated AS occurring in the adult is thought to be the result of degeneration of an abnormal valve that has functioned reasonably well for many years. Reparative techniques are usually applicable in infants, small children and young adults. Calcified, stenotic aortic valves are optimally treated by valve replacement. In infants and children, AS may involve multiple levels of the left ventricular outflow tract. In addition, congenital AS presenting in childhood is often associated with aortic annular hypoplasia. Finally, there may be additional obstructive lesions throughout the left heart.

Aortic Valve Stenosis

The surgical approach to severe congenital valvular AS in infants and children was historically based on the age and size of the patient. Early techniques involved blind dilatation or rapidly performed direct dilatation under inflow occlusion. As techniques for direct cardiac surgery on newborns evolved, precise surgical repair of AS became possible in virtually all infants and children with anatomy suitable for repair [1, 6, 9]. Percutaneous balloon aortic valvuloplasty was introduced in the mid-1980s. That technique has evolved into an effective and durable treatment for isolated valvar AS [10]. The percutaneous technique sometimes produces important aortic regurgitation (AR) and may lead to earlier valve replacement or an operation to repair the valve [2, 3]. At the present time, most patients with isolated valvar AS are treated by balloon dilatation without considering the potential benefit of a surgical approach (surgery rarely results in important early AR or compromise of a peripheral artery [7]. Since multiple levels of obstruction can be dealt with at the time of surgical aortic valvotomy, surgery is generally reserved for those patients with multi-level obstruction.

Supravalvular Aortic Stenosis

Supravalvular AS may be discrete or diffuse. The aortic arch and origins of other major arteries may also be stenotic. This entity may be associated with Williams syndrome, or it may occur as an isolated defect involving the supravalvular ascending aorta. In the usual form, there is an obvious waist at the level of the sinotubular ridge. When the aorta is opened, a ridge of tissue circumferentially obstructs the aorta at the level of the sinotubular ridge. Resection and patching of the aorta eliminates the obstruction. The initial surgical incision crosses the area of narrowing and extends into the non-coronary sinus of Valsalva. The patch may extend into one, two or all three sinuses. Severe supravalvular AS is optimally treated using the triple patch technique of Brom [4]. The aortic valve in this condition is usually trileaflet and competent. The fibrous tissue and constriction may obstruct the coronary arteries. These patients must be very carefully evaluated. Sudden death has occurred in severe cases. When the triple patch operation is utilized, late reoperation is rarely necessary.

Subaortic Stenosis

The most common type of subaortic stenosis is a fibrous ring found just below the aortic valve. The ring is generally discrete and clearly separate from the aortic valve. In some cases, the fibrous tissue extends up to the valve annulus. Rarely, it may actually extend onto the ventricular side of the valve leaflet. Operation is performed through the aortic valve. In the past, surgical resection by cutting the ring from the adjacent structures was associated with a relatively high recurrence rate of 10–15%. Most surgeons now agree that discrete subaortic stenosis is optimally treated by an enucleation technique. Enucleation peels the fibrous tissue from the septum and the leaflets. After enucleation there is often no residual fibrous tissue visible and the recurrence rate is much lower. In patients with a very hypertrophic septum, a septal myotomy or myomectomy may also be useful.

Complex forms of subaortic stenosis can involve a fibrous tunnel, which is not amenable to direct resection or enucleation. The sub-annular Konno technique is useful in the treatment of tunnel subaortic stenosis [5, 11]. In this approach, a right ventriculotomy permits creation of a ventricular septal defect. The incision in the septum is guided by a clamp placed through the normal or relatively normal aortic valve. Obstructing muscle and fibrous tissue in the subaortic region can be resected under direct vision. The surgically created ventricular septal defect is then closed with a Gore-Tex or pericardial patch.

Associated lesions such as valvar AS, supravalvar mitral ring, congenital mitral valve stenosis, and ascending aortic hypoplasia can also be repaired during the operation for subaortic stenosis. Some patients will also have coarctation of the aorta, which is usually treated by a separate procedure. The order and timing of treatment for multiple levels of obstruction in the left heart is dependent upon the severity of the associated lesions.

Critical Aortic Stenosis in the Neonate

In neonates presenting with critical AS, a decision must be made whether the left ventricle (LV) is suitable for a biventricular repair. These infants may be dependent upon their ductus arteriosus for systemic perfusion. The LV may be too small or poorly functioning. Balloon aortic valvuloplasty allows assessment of ventricular function and permits planning the appropriate definitive repair approach. When the LV is not suitable for a biventricular repair, the Norwood approach allows palliation and treatment as a functional single ventricle [8]. Cardiac transplantation may also be an option.

Repair versus the Ross Procedure in Infants and Children

In infants and small children, the suitability for repair must be assessed within the context of the possibility of the Ross operation. Since most aortic valve repair operations will ultimately be followed by aortic valve replacement, an approach which preserves the pulmonary valve for future use must be considered. In addition, the Ross operation will not be curative in infants and small children. At the minimum, an infant undergoing the Ross operation will require reoperation to replace the pulmonary homograft. Thus, a case can be made for initial palliation by aortic valve repair, unless a sub-annular Konno operation or repair of an associated ventricular septal defect might result in suturing near the pulmonary annulus (interfering with later use of the pulmonary valve).

LV outlet obstruction may occur in patients for whom the Ross procedure is not an option. In such patients, the value of repair must be assessed in comparison to the consequences of implantation of a mechanical valve. Lifestyle considerations also enter into the repair/replace decision-making process as children enter the teenage years. Some patients and their families may be unhappy with the restrictions placed upon them by residual abnormalities following repair operations. In such cases, an early Ross procedure may be performed as a means to achieve optimal exercise tolerance and freedom from anticoagulation. When the Ross procedure is not possible, an extensive repair may permit a more athletic lifestyle without the risk of anticoagulation.

In summary, LV outlet obstruction is generally amenable to repair in infants, children and young adults. When the valve is calcified, as in older patients, repair is unlikely to provide durable relief of obstruction. The timing and type of operation will be determined by the patient's age, sex, and lifestyle preferences. Repair is often the best option for young patients unsuitable for the Ross operation. While repair does not restore 'normal anatomy and function', it can provide excellent palliation for many years.

References

1 Caspi J, Ilbawi MN, Roberson DA, Piccione W, Monson DO, Najafi H: Extended aortic valvuloplasty for recurrent valvular stenosis and regurgitation in children. J Thorac Cardiovasc Surg 1994;107:1114–1120.

2 Hawkins JA, Minich LL, Tani LY, Day RW, Judd VE, Shaddy RE, McGough EC: Late results and reintervention after aortic valvotomy for critical aortic stenosis in neonates and infants. Ann Thorac Surg 1998;65:1758–1763.

3 Hawkins JA, Minich LL, Shaddy RE, Tani LY, Orsmond GS, Sturtevant JE, McGough EC: Aortic valve repair and replacement after balloon aortic valvuloplasty in children. Ann Thorac Surg 1996;61:1355–1358.

4 Hazekamp MG, Kappetein A, Schoof PH, Ottenkamp J, Witsenburg M, Huysmans HA, Bogers A: Brom's three-patch technique for repair of supravalvular aortic stenosis. J Thorac Cardiovasc Surg 1999;118:252–258.

5 Jahangiri M, Nicholson IA, Del Nido PJ, Mayer JE, Jonas RA: Surgical management of complex and tunnel-like subaortic stenosis. Eur J Cardiothorac Surg 2000;17:637–642.

6 Keane JF, Driscoll DJ, Gersony WM, Hayes CJ, Kidd L, O'Fallon WM, Pieroni DR, Wolfe RR, Weidman WH: Second natural history study of congenital heart defects, results of treatment of patients with aortic valvar stenosis. Circulation 1993;87(suppl I):16–27.

7 Lamberti JJ: The aortic valve: To dilate, repair or replace – that is the question. Ann Thorac Surg 1996;61:1297–1298.

8 Lofland GK, McCrindle BW, Williams WG, Blackstone EH, Tchervenkov CI, Sittiwangkul R, Jonas RA: Critical aortic stenosis in the neonate: A multi-institutional study of management, outcomes and risk factors. J Thorac Cardiovasc Surg 2001;121:10–27.

9 Rao V, Van Arsdell GS, David TE, Azakie A, Williams WG: Aortic valve repair for adult congenital heart disease. Circulation 2000;102(suppl III):40–43.

10 Rosenfeld HM, Landzberg MJ, Perry SB, Colan SD, Keane JF, Lock JE: Balloon aortic valvuloplasty in the young adult with congenital aortic stenosis. Am J Cardiol 1994;73:1112–1117.

11 Roughneen PT, Deleon SY, Cetta F, Vitullo DA, Bell TJ, Fisher EA, Blakeman BP, Bakhos M: Modified Konno-Rastan procedure for subaortic stenosis: Indications, operative techniques and results. Ann Thorac Surg 1998;65:1368–1376.

John J. Lamberti, MD, Department of Cardiothoracic Surgery, New York Presbyterian Hospital, New York Weill Cornell Medical Center, 525 East 68th Street, New York, NY 10021 (USA)

Borer JS, Isom OW (eds): Pathophysiology, Evaluation and Management of Valvular Heart Diseases.
Adv Cardiol. Basel, Karger, 2002, vol 39, pp 74–85

Aortic Regurgitation: Selection of Asymptomatic Patients for Valve Surgery

Jeffrey S. Borer, Edmund McM. Herrold, Clare A. Hochreiter, Phyllis G. Supino, Andrew Yin, Karl H. Krieger, O. Wayne Isom

Division of Cardiovascular Pathophysiology, Department of Cardiothoracic Surgery and The Howard Gilman Institute for Valvular Heart Diseases, Weill Medical College of Cornell University, New York, N.Y., USA

During the past two decades, criteria for aortic valve surgery have evolved gradually but substantially for patients with hemodynamically severe aortic regurgitation (AR). The changes have resulted primarily from two factors. First, surgical techniques and materials have improved considerably during this interval. Advances in prosthesis design and durability, in myocardial preservation methods, etc., have minimized surgical risks and improved long-term benefits. Second, continually evolving objective testing techniques, evaluation algorithms and comparator databases have enhanced prognostic accuracy, enabling identification of subsets of asymptomatic patients who are at relatively high risk of untoward event if operation is not performed, justifying operation for reasons other than symptom relief alone.

The Symptomatic Patient: Incomplete Knowledge

Development of symptoms of any severity now is considered a primary indication for operation. Until 25 years ago, symptoms needed to reach New York Heart Association (NYHA) Functional Class III (i.e., occurring during less than 'normal' activity) before operation was indicated in the judgment of most cardiologists. At the time, relief of symptoms of this severity by surgery was predictable but often incomplete. Concomitant short- and long-term risks of operation were high relative to current expectations, and were considered inordinate when measured against the frequent lack of symptomatic improvement when symptoms were of lesser severity (and when enhanced survival could not be inferred confidently after surgery). Moreover, the natural history of the symptomatic patient was not precisely defined because objective measures were not routinely performed until immediately prior to surgery. Nonetheless, available data suggested that patients with clear congestive symptoms and AR were at higher mortality risk than those without symptoms. Therefore, it was hoped that valve replacement would improve survival while relieving symptoms.

Today, operation generally produces symptom reduction or relief even for those with relatively modest limitation in activity tolerance. This benefit may relate to improving myocardial preservation techniques, hemodynamically more effective prostheses, etc. However, dependence on symptom development as the sole indication for surgery brings with it several problems. First, it can be difficult to define and, therefore, to identify symptoms. Symptoms are subjective complaints and their quantification is ambiguous. Symptoms that qualify as NYHA Functional Class III (or worse) are relatively unequivocal: they involve perceptible dyspnea and/or fatigue during activity of less than 'normal' intensity and generally (but not always) are recognized as causing important changes in lifestyle. Lesser symptoms can be harder to identify. Functional Class II symptoms occur with activity that is 'normal' in intensity. Does this mean that dyspnea after two flights of stairs represents evidence of heart failure when a trip of this magnitude is taken only twice a year, even though it could be achieved a few years ago? How does the physician account for the suggestibility of a patient who knows that he or she has valvular disease, that this may cause symptoms and that failure to report the symptoms may result in inappropriate medical decisions? The physician, too, may be susceptible to such unintentional interpretation bias. Indeed, as noted below, in our recent study of the importance of contractility measurement in prognostication among asymptomatic or 'minimally' symptomatic patients [1], we found that, at index study, 18 patients reported diminution in exercise tolerance compared with the previous year. However, their absolute activity levels were within what generally would be accepted as a normal range. The following year, these 18 patients no longer reported the limitation, a fact not reported in the publication (the primary analysis was focused only on patient condition at study entry). Since the NYHA system provides no classification for such patients, they were reported in the publication as being in 'Early Functional Class II' (also denoted as 'Class I to II' in the interview notes) at index study. However, if the report had been based on the interview performed the following year, they would have been included in Functional Class I. Four additional patients reported complaints that were not clearly of cardiac origin and were listed similarly (though these patients may, indeed, truly have had subtle early Functional Class II symptoms based on a cardiac cause). Thus, though recent studies suggest that symptoms represent a major risk factor for clinical and LV functional deterioration and death, and the clear development of symptoms almost universally is accepted as an indication for operation, agreement on what constitutes such symptoms may be less complete.

The result has been increasing dependence on objective measures of LV size and function for decisions about management of patients with AR. When some of these measures (particularly those obtained with the patient at rest) become abnormal, symptoms often occur at approximately the same time. However, concordance is far from complete between symptom development and objective abnormalities. Indeed, when symptoms are associated with LV dysfunction at rest, relatively poor survival can be expected even if operation is performed [2]. No randomized trials of surgery versus nonsurgical management have been performed among symptomatic patients with AR. Therefore, it is impossible to assert rigorously that aortic valve replacement (AVR) improves survival in these patients, though inferences from early surgical series suggest such benefit [3] when compared with published natural history assessments of unoperated symptomatic patients [18], while nonrandomized observational data report maintenance of normal survival patterns when symptomatic and asymptomatic patients undergo AVR before specific indices of myocardial deterioration are apparent [4]. Given the limitations of the knowledge base for management decisions in symptomatic patients, the controversy surrounding surgery for the asymptomatic patient is not surprising.

The Asymptomatic Patient

The natural history of the asymptomatic patient with AR and normal left ventricular ejection fraction (LVEF) at rest has been defined in several studies involving as many as 104 patients followed for as long as 15 years. Absolute progression rates vary modestly among these studies, probably reflecting minor differences in selection factors, population size and duration of follow-up. Nonetheless, the numbers are remarkably similar: except for a very small early study suggesting progression to symptoms at a rate of 9%/year [2], published progression rates range from about 4 to 6%/year [1, 5–7] for development of congestive symptoms, subnormal LVEF at rest, or sudden death (fig. 1). Moreover, progression to endpoints tends to be linear, without evidence of significant increase as time after diagnosis lengthens.

A firm consensus has not been reached on appropriate criteria for undertaking aortic valve surgery in an asymptomatic patient with AR, though The American College of Cardiology has provided a very useful review and inclusive set of considerations [8]. Nonetheless, reasonably persuasive data support

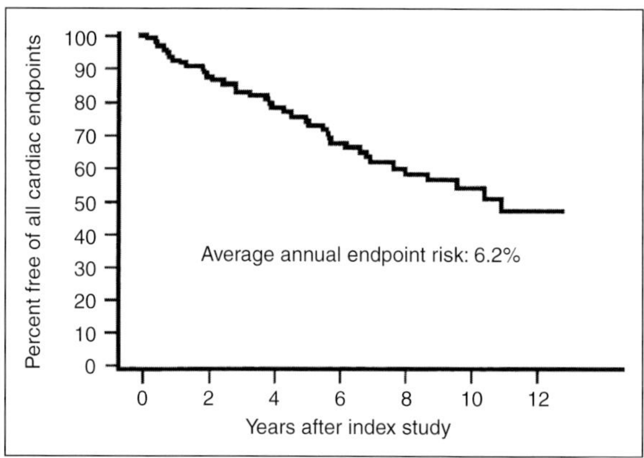

Fig. 1. Natural history of progression to endpoints in severe chronic AR [from 1, with permission].

three primary criteria: (1) subnormal LV performance/function while the patient is at rest, (2) relatively marked LV dilatation at rest and (3) marked LV dysfunction induced by exercise even in the absence of criteria 1 and 2.

Subnormal LV Performance/Function While the Patient Is at Rest

LV performance or function can be estimated by ejection fraction (EF) obtained by contrast angiography at catheterization, by radionuclide angiography, by echocardiography or by magnetic resonance imaging. Intrinsic myocardial function, or contractility, can be measured more precisely by adjusting LVEF, a performance descriptor, for extrinsic loading conditions [1, 9, 10, 17]. Contractility measures include wall stress-adjusted EF [1], pressure volume index [9, 10, 17], or ventricular elastance (obtained by invasive or noninvasive methods, or by combinations of these approaches) [11].

If LVEF, or any other measure of LV function, is subnormal at rest in an asymptomatic patient and symptoms then develop, the patient will be at relatively high risk for irreversible heart failure or death until AVR is performed. In addition, at this relatively late stage in the natural history of AR, long-term survival (and, to some extent, symptom relief) will be disappointing even if AVR is performed [2]. However, when LVEF is subnormal at rest in the asymptomatic patient, progression to symptoms is predictably rapid, occurring at a rate of 25%/year [12]. Thus, when LVEF is subnormal at rest, the imminent development of symptoms and, therefore, the imminent need for operation that is likely to produce suboptimal benefit, can be predicted with reasonable confidence. Consequently, operation before the development of symptoms seems justified.

Table 1. Relation of LV FS at rest to development of congestive heart (CHF) during follow-up in patients with AR [modified from 2, with permission]

Echo %FS	Index study	CHF during F/U (mean 34 months)	CHF development rate %/year estimate
Normal	28	8 (29%)	<9
Subnormal	9	6 (67%)	>25

Echo = Echocardiogram.

The data from which these conclusions are drawn were developed more than 20 years ago in two studies that included a relatively small number of patients (table 1) [2, 12]. In the first, among 49 patients with symptomatic AR who underwent AVR, those whose echocardiographic fractional shortening (FS) was normal at rest before operation manifested a 5-year post-operative survival in excess of 90%, while only 60% survived 5 years when pre-operative FS was subnormal. The second study, and still the primary basis for operation in asymptomatic patients with subnormal LV function at rest, involved 37 patients, 28 of whom manifested normal FS at rest at their index study. The study was published before many of current statistical methods and modes of data presentation were regularly applied to evaluate survival data; precise progression rates were not presented and cannot be defined post-hoc from the published data. Nonetheless, review of these data suggests that heart failure developed in these asymptomatic patients at a rate of approximately 9%/year, higher than was found by later, larger and longer studies (perhaps because these later studies generally excluded patients with subnormal LVEF/FS at rest). Among the 9 patients whose LV FS was subnormal at study entry despite the absence of symptoms, 6, or two-thirds, developed heart failure during follow-up; the rate of heart failure development in these patients was slightly greater than 25%/year.

Clearly, these data provide an incomplete understanding of the natural history of the asymptomatic patient with subnormal LVEF at rest. Among patients with subnormal FS, the duration of impaired LV function was unknown at study entry, the study population was small relative to current standards and measurements were made by M-mode echocardiography, without the benefit of direction by two-dimensional imaging, developed shortly thereafter. Nonetheless, rate of symptom development in the sub-cohort with impaired LV function was sufficiently rapid, the results of operation in these and similar populations were sufficiently disappointing and, intuitively, the study results were sufficiently reasonable so that additional data are not likely to be collected to clarify natural history after LV function is subnormal at rest. Therefore, on the basis of these data, it is widely accepted that the peri-operative and long-term risks of AVR in asymptomatic patients with subnormal LVEF at rest are considerably less than the risks of not operating. Surgical methods have improved over the years since the study was performed, though the natural history of the unoperated patient is unlikely to have improved substantially (despite the controversial use of vasodilating drugs, dihydropyridine calcium channel blockers or angiotensin-converting enzyme inhibitors and angiotensin receptor blockers in some of these patients). Consequently, over time, the relative advantage of AVR probably has increased for the asymptomatic patient with subnormal LV function at rest.

Marked LV Dilatation at Rest

LV dilatation can be defined both in systole and in diastole. Systolic dilatation, as a 'systolic phase index', is a reflection of LV function and myocardial contractility. Indeed, marked systolic dilatation, manifested as echocardiographic LV internal dimension in systole (LVIDs) >55 mm, predicts post-operative survival and symptom development as well as or better than FS, and remains a persuasive basis for operation in the asymptomatic patient [2, 12]. However, relatively few data support operation for diastolic LV dilatation. Nonetheless, marked diastolic dilatation provides a plausible basis for deterioration of myocardial function, since LV wall stress throughout systole, the putative mechanical initiator of intrinsic myocardial damage, increases as a function of the dimension at which systole begins, that is, end-diastole. Concern regarding diastolic dilatation was stimulated by the anecdotal reports of 2 sudden deaths among a small number of patients with echocardiographic LVID in diastole (d) >80 mm [13] and sporadic other anecdotes suggesting that risk pertains at LVID ⩾75 mm. However, the best argument for 'prophylactic' valve replacement in patients with marked LV dilatation is the observation that, irrespective of symptoms, long-term post operative survival among 31 patients who underwent AVR with LVIDd ⩾80 mm was significantly poorer than that of the unselected age-matched US population from census data (presumably including only a small proportion of individuals with AR), while post-operative survival of patients with LVIDd below this cutpoint was not significantly different from that of the census-derived population [4]. When matched against each other, survival of the more and less dilated groups was *not* statistically distinguishable. Also, LVEF was found to be a significant predictor of survival in the study population. Nonetheless, these data suggest that LVIDd >80 mm independently identifies patients whose long-term prognosis has begun to deteriorate and who are likely to benefit progressively less from operation if AVR is further delayed.

The magnitude of risk among asymptomatic patients with LVIDd ⩾80 mm cannot be defined from the available data. Only a modest number of patients provided data for construction of survival curves for each LVIDd-based subset.

The resulting variability of these data renders point estimates of risk relatively unstable. Nonetheless, as in the case of subnormal LVEF at rest, a relative advantage of operation in the patient with marked diastolic dilatation seems reasonable to infer. The appropriate cutpoint is less clear. The 80-mm criterion is drawn from a moderately sized study designed to evaluate the importance of LV dilatation; the 75-mm criterion is based on anecdotes that establish an arguable case for the more stringent criterion, since the outcome in these cases was sudden death. However, perhaps the issue can be resolved by application of the third criterion, an abnormality induced by exercise.

Markedly Subnormal Contractility Unmasked by Exercise

Intuitively, it seems reasonable that LV dysfunction induced by stress, but not present at rest, must represent an intermediate point between normal LV function and LV dysfunction apparent even at rest. Indeed, the validity of this concept seemed clear from the earliest studies of LVEF response to exercise in patients with AR, more than 20 years ago [14]. However, demonstration of the prognostic value of exercise-induced dysfunction required an additional 20 years of study, involving prolonged follow-up of a relatively large population and the development of methods to allow reasonably precise contractility measures from noninvasive data obtained during exercise, when accuracy of geometric measures can be confounded by patient motion [14].

To obtain the necessary contractility data, 104 patients underwent testing with both radionuclide cineangiography, at rest and during maximal supine bicycle exercise, and echocardiography at rest, at entry into a prospective epidemiological study [1]. In order to be included in subsequent analyses, all patients needed to manifest normal LVEF at rest. They were generally totally asymptomatic, in that they had no difficulty performing their normal activities. However, as noted previously, some perceived changes in their effort tolerance from earlier years and some reported exercise 'limitations' that subsequently were absent despite the fact that no treatment had been applied.

To determine contractility, LVEF change (Δ) from rest to exercise was adjusted for change in end-systolic wall stress (ΔLVESS; LVESS is an accepted measure of LV afterload) from rest to exercise. While the former parameter could be defined easily with radionuclide cineangiography, the stress parameter required combination of echocardiographic and radionuclide ventriculographic data, employing appropriate adjustments and assumptions drawn from the physics of mechanics. An index of contractility was constructed by determining the relation of ΔLVEF and ΔESS among a cohort of normal subjects, and then defining the extent to which ΔLVEF in a patient varied from the value expected in a normal subject operating at the patient's ΔESS (fig. 2). Patients then were categorized as to their contractility index (and also by the results of the other measures of

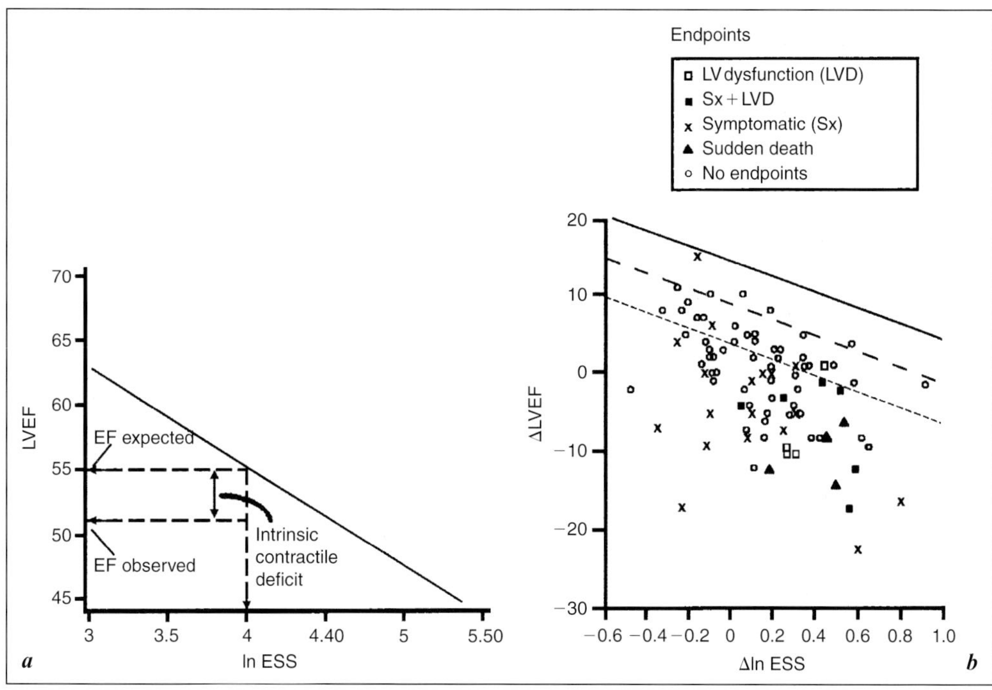

Fig. 2. ***a*** Relation of a performance descriptor, LVEF, to a loading descriptor, end-systolic stress (ESS), after log transformation (ln) of ESS, as defined from 26 normal subjects. To define LVEF-ESS index for a patient, patient's ln ESS is determined and, from normal regression line, expected LVEF is defined. Patient's measured LVEF (EF observed) is then subtracted from expected value. Difference is LVEF-ESS index. ***b*** Relation of ΔLVEF to Δln ESS, analogous to relation depicted in ***a***, for 88 patients with severe AR. Solid regression line defines this relation in 26 normal subjects; dashed lines represent 1 and 2 SD below this mean normal relation. Clinical outcome (endpoints) in patients is defined by symbols, as noted [from 1, with permission].

LV performance and geometry (i.e., ΔLVEF, EF rest, EF exercise, LVIDd, LVIDs, FS, LV mass, etc.) that were made in the context of providing the raw data for contractility determinations.

When analyzed according to contractility, development of symptoms, of subnormal LVEF at rest, or of sudden death, could be predicted with high statistical significance. In fact, though other parameters also showed predictive value, the contractility index was the strongest independent predictor of outcome. (The closest imitator was ΔLVEF, alone, unadjusted for stress; this measure also was highly predictive of outcome events, though not quite so strong as intrinsic contractility.) As seen in figure 1, in this study population, endpoints developed at

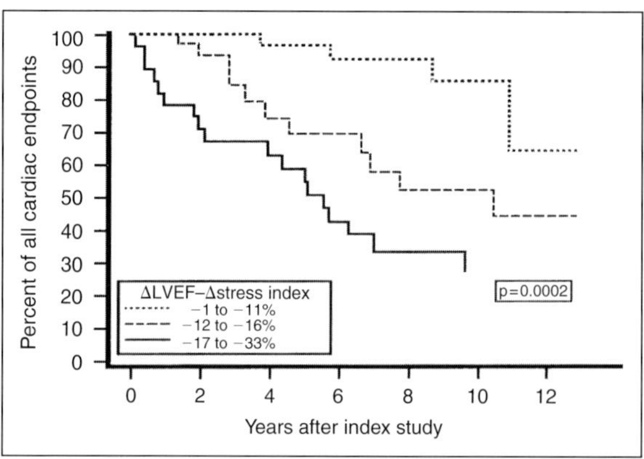

Fig. 3. Relation of ΔLVEF-ΔESS index at study entry to occurrence of any cardiac endpoint (cardiac death, operable symptoms, and/or subnormal LV performance at rest) during follow-up. Population of 88 patients with evaluable data for this analysis has been divided statistically into terciles. ΔLVEF-ΔESS index boundaries for each tercile are boxed [from 1, with permission].

a rate of approximately 6%/year. However, when the full cohort was subdivided into equal terciles based on contractility, the third with the highest contractility at baseline progressed to endpoints at a rate of 1.8%/year (fig. 3). In contrast, the third with the poorest contractility at baseline, despite normal LVEF at rest, progressed at a rate almost 10 times faster, that is, approximately 15%/year, while the middle third developed endpoints at a rate midway between those of the polar extremes. In other words, within 3 years, almost half the patients with particularly subnormal contractility can be expected to develop accepted criteria for AVR, or to die suddenly. The relation of contractility to outcome was true not only for all endpoints considered together, but also for the individual endpoints of congestive symptoms and/or subnormal LVEF at rest. However, sudden death occurred *only* in those with markedly subnormal contractility; this catastrophic outcome occurred at a rate of approximately 1%/year in this subgroup. The sudden death data are particularly striking. Though anecdotes had been reported previously, this was the first time that a statistically significant predictor of sudden death, alone, had been identified for AR. It is plausible that the distinction between LVIDd of 75 versus 80 mm as a criterion for AVR can be resolved with reference to contractility data obtained during exercise (an assessment not previously performed in studies of patients with AR). To resolve this issue, we reviewed the data for the 98 patients in our study population for whom LVIDd was available. Sudden death occurred in 1 patient among the 17 who had LVIDd ≥75 mm; in this patient, LVIDd was 78 mm. No deaths occurred in the

10 patients with LVIDd ⩾80 mm (range 80–87 mm). The remaining 3 sudden deaths occurred among patients with LVIDd <75 mm. Thus, sudden death rates among those with LVIDd ⩾75 mm were indistinguishable from those with smaller diastolic dimensions in this patient set, while contractility clearly differentiated those at relatively high risk of sudden death.

Most importantly, however, the identification of sudden death as a predictable endpoint in asymptomatic patients with AR adds great impetus to the application of criteria for AVR based on prognostically important objective changes that occur before development of symptoms. As yet, of course, no data have demonstrated a reduction in sudden death rate associated with AVR performed at any point in the natural history of the disease. Nonetheless, with the progressively improving survival among patients with AR who undergo AVR, it is highly likely that operation does provide life-prolonging benefits, with sudden death reduction, when applied before development of severe LV dysfunction, either at rest or unmasked by exercise.

Finally, even if patients did not achieve the high-risk contractility descriptor at study entry, relatively poor prognosis could be inferred if ΔLVEF deteriorated particularly rapidly over time [15]. Application of this finding in selecting patients for operation requires additional study.

As is true for the other criteria presented herein for operation among asymptomatic patients, the contractility index criterion is based on relatively few data and only one study. However, this finding has been buttressed by the preliminary observation that the same contractility index is the best predictor of long-term post-operative survival after AVR, and is considerably better than resting measures of LV performance and geometry [16]. Thus, there is considerable reason to accept this criterion as a particularly sensitive means of identifying patients who will benefit from 'prophylactic' operation. Nonetheless, a cautionary note is appropriate: all objective tests involve a certain magnitude of methodological variability, which is confounded by some degree of biological variability. Therefore, before applying an objective measure as a basis for operation in an asymptomatic patient, repetition of the test should be undertaken and directional and, perhaps, amplitude concordance among the results should be sought.

Conclusion

The most universally accepted basis for operation in patients with AR is the development of symptoms. If nothing else, AVR can be expected to make the patient feel better. However, when symptoms have occurred, long-term prognosis, with or without operation, already is importantly compromised.

Therefore, operation in the asymptomatic patient must be seriously considered. Though data from rigorous contemporaneous comparisons of management strategies have not been performed, available data suggest that the risk : benefit ratio of operating is likely to support pre-symptomatic operation if LVEF already is subnormal at rest, if marked (>80 mm) LV dilatation has occurred, or if markedly subnormal LV contractility is unmasked by exercise. Additional study is needed to define precisely the predictive value of results obtained with any of these approaches and to supplement or modify the suggested criteria with reference to collateral data.

Acknowledgements

Dr. Borer is the Gladys and Roland Harriman Professor of Cardiovascular Medicine at Cornell and was supported in part during this work by an endowment from the Gladys and Roland Harriman Foundation, New York, N.Y. In addition, the work reported herein was supported in part by National Heart Lung and Blood Institute, Bethesda, Md. (RO1-HL-26504), and by grants from The Howard Gilman Foundation, New York, N.Y., The Schiavone Family Foundation, White House Station, N.J., The Charles and Jean Brunie Foundation, Bronxville, N.Y., The David Margolis Foundation, New York, N.Y., The American Cardio-Vascular Research Foundation, New York, N.Y., The Irving R. Hansen Foundation, New York, N.Y., The Mary A.H. Rumsey Foundation, New York, N.Y., The Messinger Family Foundation, New York, N.Y., The Daniel and Elaine Sargent Charitable Trust, New York, N.Y., The A.C. Israel Foundation, Greenwich, Conn., and by much appreciated gifts from Maryjane and the late William Voute, Bronxville, N.Y., and Stephen and Suzanne Weiss, Greenwich, Conn.

References

1 Borer JS, Hochreiter C, Herrold EM, Supino P, Aschermann M, Wencker D, Devereux RB, Roman MJ, Szulc M, Kligfield P, Isom OW: Prediction of indications for valve replacement among asymptomatic or minimally symptomatic patients with chronic aortic regurgitation and normal left ventricular performance. Circulation 1998;97:525–534.
2 Henry WL, Bonow RO, Borer JS, Ware JH, Kent KM, Redwood DR, McIntosh CL, Morrow AG, Epstein SE: Observations on the optimum time for operative intervention for aortic regurgitation. I. Evaluation of the results of aortic valve replacement in symptomatic patients. Circulation 1980;61:471–483.
3 Samuels DA, Curfman GD, Friedlich AL, Buckley MJ, Austen WG: Valve replacement for aortic regurgitation: Long-term follow-up with factors influencing the results. Circulation 1979;60: 647–654.
4 Klodas E, Enriquez-Sarano M, Tajik AJ, Mullany CJ, Bailey KR, Seward JB: Aortic regurgitation complicated by extreme left ventricular dilation: Long-term outcome after surgical correction. J Am Coll Cardiol 1996;27:670–677.
5 Bonow RO, Rosing DR, McIntosh CL, Jones M, Maron BJ, Lan KKG, Lakatos E, Bacharach SL, Green MV, Epstein SE: The natural history of asymptomatic patients with aortic regurgitation and normal left ventricular function. Circulation 1983;68:509–517.
6 Siemienczuk D, Greenberg B, Morris C, Massie B, Wilson RA, Topic N, Bristow JD, Cheitlin M: Chronic aortic insufficiency: Factors associated with progression to aortic valve replacement. Ann Intern Med 1989;110:587–592.

7 Greves J, Rahimtoola SH, McAnulty JH, DeMots H, Clark DG, Greenberg B, Starr A: Preoperative criteria predictive of late survival following valve replacement for severe aortic regurgitation. Am Heart J 1981;101:300–308.

8 Bonow RO, Carabello B, de Leon AC Jr, Edmunds LH Jr, Fedderly BJ, Freed MD, Gaasch WH, McKay CR, Nishimura RA, O'Gara PT, O'Rourke RA, Rahimtoola SH, Ritchie JL, Cheitlin MD, Eagle KA, Gardner TJ, Garson A Jr, Gibbons RJ, Russell RO, Ryan TJ, Smith SC Jr: Guidelines for the management of patients with valvular heart disease: Executive summary. A report of the American College of Cardiology/American Heart Association Task Force on Practice Guidelines (Committee on Management of Patients with Valvular Heart Disease). Circulation 1998;18: 1949–1984.

9 Carabello BA, Williams H, Gash AK, Kent R, Belber D, Maurer A, Siegel J, Blasius K, Spann JF: Hemodynamic predictors of outcome in patients undergoing valve replacement. Circulation 1986;74:1309–1316.

10 Wisenbaugh T, Booth D, DeMaria A, Nissen S, Waters J: Relationship of contractile state to ejection performance in patients with chronic aortic valve disease. Circulation 1986;73:47–53.

11 Shen FW, Roubin GS, Choong CYP, Hutton BF, Harris PJ, Fletcher PJ, Kelly DT: Evaluation of the relationship between myocardial contractile state and left ventricular function in patients with aortic regurgitation. Circulation 1985;71:1–38.

12 Henry WL, Bonow RO, Rosing DR, Epstein SE: Observations on the optimum time for operative intervention for aortic regurgitation. II. Serial echocardiographic evaluation of asymptomatic patients. Circulation 1980;61:484–492.

13 Bonow RO, Lakatos E, Maron BJ, Epstein ES: Serial long-term assessment of the natural history of asymptomatic patients with chronic aortic regurgitation and normal left ventricular systolic function. Circulation 1991;84:1625–1635.

14 Borer JS, Bacharach SL, Green MV, Kent KM, Henry WL, Rosing DR, Seides SF, Johnston GS, Epstein SE: Exercise-induced left ventricular dysfunction in symptomatic and asymptomatic patients with aortic regurgitation: Assessment by radionuclide cineangiography. Am J Cardiol 1978;42:351–357.

15 Supino PG, Borer JS, Hochreiter C, Herrold EM, Kligfield P, Devereux RB, Roman MJ: Chronic aortic regurgitation: Natural history of rest and exercise ejection fraction and relation to outcome (abstract). Circulation 1999;100(suppl I):519.

16 Borer JS, Hochreiter C, Herrold EM, Roman MJ, Kligfield P, Szulc M, Supino P, Isom OW, Krieger K, Kaufman JD: Prediction of outcome late after aortic valve replacement for aortic regurgitation utilizing pre-operative wall-stress-adjusted change in ejection fraction from rest to exercise (abstract). Circulation 1998;98(suppl I):475.

17 Gaasch WH, Carroll JD, Levine HJ, Criscitiello MG: Chronic aortic regurgitation: Prognostic value of left ventricular end-diastolic radius/thickness ratio. J Am Coll Cardiol 1983;1:775–782.

18 Braunwald EB: Valvular heart disease: Aortic regurgitation; in Braunwald EB (ed): Heart Disease: A Textbook of Cardiovascular Medicine. Philadelphia, Saunders, 1980, pp 1138–1147.

Jeffrey S. Borer, MD, Division of Cardiovascular Pathophysiology,
New York Presbyterian Hospital, New York Weill Cornell Center,
525 East 68th Street, New York, NY 10021 (USA)

Borer JS, Isom OW (eds): Pathophysiology, Evaluation and Management of Valvular Heart Diseases.
Adv Cardiol. Basel, Karger, 2002, vol 39, pp 86–92

Surgical Approaches When Aortic Regurgitation Is Associated with Aortic Root Disease

Leonard N. Girardi

Department of Cardiothoracic Surgery, and The Howard Gilman Institute for Valvular Heart Diseases, Weill Medical College of Cornell University, New York-Presbyterian Hospital-New York Weill Cornell Medical Center, New York, N.Y., USA

Surgery for aortic insufficiency in the setting of aortic root disease is more complex than isolated aortic valve replacement. Extensive aortic root reconstruction may be required in patients with bicuspid aortic valves, supravalvular stenosis or in the setting of destructive native or prosthetic valve endocarditis. A majority of patients, however, have annuloaortic ectasia and an ascending aortic aneurysm. This may be associated with severe atherosclerosis, long-standing hypertension, acute or chronic aortic dissection or an inflammatory aneurysm [1–3]. The largest category of patients with this disease continues to be those with connective tissue disorders such as Marfan's syndrome, Ehlers-Danlos syndrome or patients with familial aneurysm and dissection syndromes [4]. A variety of surgical techniques have been developed that eliminate the risk of aortic dissection and aortic rupture while providing relief from aortic valve insufficiency. Traditional techniques involve replacement of the aorta with a synthetic graft and aortic valve replacement with either a mechanical or bioprosthesis. This can be accomplished as two separate components or as a single unit, composite valve graft. Cadaveric, homograft aortic root replacement accomplishes the same goal and may be beneficial in specific circumstances. Finally, preservation of the native aortic valve, in the setting of ascending aortic aneurysm repair, may also be worthwhile for certain individuals. This review will outline the indications for aortic root reconstruction and the surgical techniques involved. In addition to the perioperative mortality and morbidity of the various procedures, intermediate and long-term expectations will also be outlined. The option of aortic root reconstruction with a pulmonary autograft, the Ross procedure, both with and without

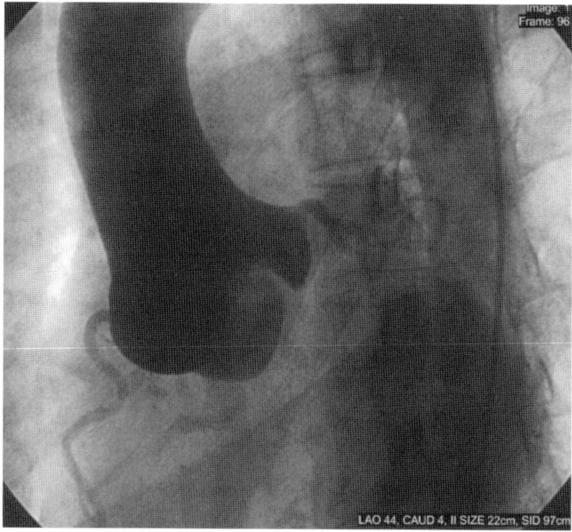

Fig. 1. Aortogram of a patient with an ascending aortic aneurysm with a connective tissue disorder. The sinuses of Valsalva are markedly dilated, and the coronary arteries are effaced high into their respective sinuses. The remainder of the ascending aorta is of relatively normal diameter.

annular reduction techniques, is presented elsewhere in this volume and will not be discussed further [5, 6].

Once a patient has attained an ascending aortic diameter of 5.5 cm, surgery should be performed to avoid rupture or dissection, regardless of the status of the aortic valve. Those patients with aortic growth of >1 cm/year should also be referred for elective reconstruction. Patients with unexplained chest pain syndromes, in the presence of an aneurysm of any size, should also consider surgery. In patients with a family history of dissection or rupture, surgery should be considered at aortic diameters as small as 4.5 cm. The most common etiology in patients requiring aortic root reconstruction is annuloaortic ectasia with aortic insufficiency and an aortic aneurysm (fig. 1). The annulus is markedly dilated with central aortic insufficiency. The sinuses of Valsalva are dilated, often asymmetrically, with the noncoronary sinus usually being the largest of the three. The sinotubular junction is dilated, further contributing to altered valve function. The coronary arteries are effaced, sitting quite high in their respective sinuses. They, too, may be aneurysmal and require additional surgical intervention such as coronary bypass grafting.

Nonoperative management of thoracic aortic aneurysms is associated with an extraordinarily poor short- and long-term outcome. The earliest reported natural history study of thoracic aneurysms came from the University of Hawaii, published in 1980 [7]: 157 patients were followed without surgical intervention with 5-year survival of only 20%. A similar study was published approximately one decade later. The 5-year survival in this study was 13%, with a 2-year median survival of 50% [8]. A majority of the deaths in this series were from aneurysm rupture. When an aortic dissection was the etiology of the aortic aneurysm, the survival was reduced to 7% at 5 years, while patients with atherosclerotic aneurysms had a 5-year survival of nearly 20%. Despite the introduction of aggressive hypertension management and β-blockade, a large natural history study from Scandinavia was published in 1995 with strikingly similar results [9].

When significant aortic valve regurgitation and aortic root disease coexist, a number of surgical options can be considered. The least complex procedure involves aortic valve replacement and separate replacement of the ascending aorta. A standard aortic valve replacement is performed with either a mechanical or bioprosthetic valve and a synthetic aortic graft is used to replace the ascending aorta down to the level of the sinotubular junction. The sinuses of Valsalva are left intact, or perhaps the noncoronary sinus may be excised and replaced with an extension of the aortic prosthesis down to the level of the annulus. The ascending aorta is resected in a cephalad direction to the level of the innominate artery. Not uncommonly, the dilatation of the ascending aorta extends into the proximal aortic arch, and this, too, is replaced during a brief period of profound hypothermic circulatory arrest. This procedure is technically quite simple and can be performed rapidly, and the risks of suture line bleeding are minimal. This may be the procedure of choice in elderly patients with indications for aortic valve replacement where the aortic pathology is coincidental but not the primary concern. The speed of the operation may also make it the most appropriate operation for patients with severely reduced ventricular function in which prolonged periods of myocardial ischemia may not be well tolerated. Long-term follow-up of patients undergoing separate valve and graft aortic root reconstruction reveals that approximately 15% of patients will develop aortic root aneurysms at a mean of 7–10 years post-operatively [10, 11]. Many of these recurrences are in young patients with unrecognized connective tissue disorders. These patients clearly had insufficient surgery and were inappropriate candidates for any procedure less than full root replacement. In properly selected patients, however, this should be their only operation, successfully treating both the valve and aortic pathology.

Homograft replacement of the aortic valve and ascending aorta is a less commonly performed method of treating aortic root disease and aortic insufficiency. Widespread application of this useful technique is limited by a number of factors. The greater complexity of conduit insertion, and thus the increased operative mortality, clearly deters many surgeons from incorporating this procedure into their practice. Additionally, the limited availability and high cost of homograft conduits further reduces the interest in adopting this procedure for routine use. The obvious advantages of cadaveric tissue include the avoidance of anticoagulation and the enhanced hemodynamic performance of a stentless, human valve in the aortic position. However, even with modern methods of cryopreservation [12] or with the use of fresh, 'homovital' valves [13], long-term durability remains in question. Cryopreserved conduits had an 85% freedom from failure rate at 8 years while homovital valves had slightly improved durability with an actuarial freedom from failure rate of 89% at 10 years. The actual structural valve deterioration rate is likely to be substantially higher than the actuarial data, given the relatively short mean follow-up period of only 4.8 years in this report.

Early conduit failure may be due to accelerated calcification of the aortic wall leading to leaflet degeneration. A component of immunologic rejection has also been postulated and valve durability may be improved with the use of low-dose immunosuppression. Additionally, early conduit failure is statistically more prevalent in younger patients or in donors who were <25 or >55 years of age. Thromboembolic events have not been completely avoided, and the incidence of homograft valve endocarditis is not insignificant [12, 13]. Given the enhanced durability and improved hemodynamic performance of modern bioprosthetic valves [14], the presumed advantages of homograft conduits are less obvious, further reducing their usefulness to unique situations.

In the early 1980s, Yacoub et al. [15] reported data for patients undergoing aortic valve-sparing aortic root reconstruction. They postulated that, in specific circumstances, aortic insufficiency was secondary to dilatation of the aortic sinuses and the sinotubular junction rather than primary leaflet failure. Patients could have replacement of their aorta with an artificial graft while restoring function of the native aortic valve. The procedure consists of complete resection of the ascending aorta down to the aortic annulus. Small 'buttons' of aortic tissue are left around the origins of the coronary arteries. A Dacron graft is then scalloped to recreate the sinuses of Valsalva, resuspending the native aortic valve inside the synthetic graft. The coronary arteries are then reimplanted in their proper location in the aortic root.

Since its introduction, the procedure has gained more widespread acceptance and been used in an increasing cohort of patients with marked annular dilatation, severe aortic insufficiency and even connective tissue disorders. Like homograft root replacement, the advantages of this technique are the avoidance of anticoagulation and the benefits of improved hemodynamics with the patient's native aortic valve in situ. Deterioration of the valve by calcification or low-grade rejection is not an issue. Thus, durability may be enhanced.

David et al. [16] recently published results for 120 patients undergoing aortic valve-sparing surgery. The 10-year, actuarial freedom from aortic root reoperation was an excellent 99%. However, 10-year actuarial freedom from developing moderate or severe aortic insufficiency was 83%. The actual percentage of patients having moderate to severe aortic insufficiency was 41% at a mean follow-up time of only 35 months. Additionally, the 10-year actuarial freedom from a thromboembolic event was only 89%, further reducing the attractiveness of this very technically demanding procedure. Operative mortality was low at <2%, though >10% of patients required re-exploration for bleeding in the post-operative period [17]. The best long-term results were obtained in patients who had an annular diameter of <55 mm and in those without aortic valve leaflet pathology that required leaflet reconstruction. Patients with Marfan's syndrome were also subjected to aortic valve-sparing aortic root replacement [18]. Their peri-operative mortality was slightly higher than for patients without a connective tissue disorder, 4.9%, and their actuarial freedom from reoperation at 5 years was only 83%. Perhaps the results for this operation could be improved if surgery were performed when the diameter of the annulus is closer to 50 mm and before severe valve leaflet degeneration occurs. Patients with connective tissue disorders should be made aware of the intermediate-term results of aortic valve-sparing surgery prior to proceeding. Longer follow-up is necessary before this procedure can be recommended for a less selected group of patients with aortic insufficiency.

Composite valve graft replacement of the ascending aorta and aortic valve is the gold standard operation against which all other root replacement and remodeling procedures must be compared. Developed in 1968 by Bentall and DeBono [19], this procedure immediately reduced the operative mortality for ascending aneurysm repair from nearly 20% to <10%. The original procedure consisted of a hand made composite of a prosthetic valve and a Dacron graft. This was placed inside the aortic aneurysm, the so-called inclusion graft technique, and the coronary arteries were reimplanted into the side of the ascending aortic graft. Placing the composite inside the native aorta markedly reduced the incidence of severe post-operative hemorrhage, the main cause of peri-operative death. With the advent of new valve and graft technology, numerous commercially available composite valve grafts exist, and results have continued to improve [20]. Collagen impregnation of the graft has nearly eliminated transgraft bleeding while current bileaflet, central flow, Pyrolite carbon valves have reduced the need for high levels of anticoagulation. The procedure requires meticulous attention to hemostasis but, unlike aortic valve-sparing procedures, can be learned and reproduced with a high degree of success even in emergent situations.

Multiple reports have confirmed the reliable short- and long-term results one can expect with composite valve graft replacement of the ascending aorta and aortic valve (table 1). The operative mortality is <4% in the modern surgical era. Since July 1997, we have utilized the exclusion technique [21] for our last 100 procedures, both elective and emergent cases, and have been without an operative or in-hospital mortality. Less than 4% of patients have required reoperation

Table 1. AR and aortic root disease composite valve graft

Author	Year	Cases, n	Mortality, %
Cabrol	1985	100	4.0
Lytle	1989	120	8.5
Svensson	1992	348	10.0
Kouchoukos	1992	172	5.0
Gott	1999	675	1.5
Girardi	2001	100	0

for post-operative bleeding, and nearly 60% had the procedure performed without the need for blood transfusion. No patient has required reoperation for valve or graft failure. A multicenter collection of nearly 675 composite valve grafts in Marfan's patients reports similar results [22]. The mortality for an elective procedure in this series was only 1.5% and the 10-year actuarial survival was >90%. Freedom from thromboembolism exceeded 90% at 20 years, and nearly all of these patients had complete neurologic recovery. Long-term durability was evident with only 3.4% of patients requiring reoperation on any part of their aorta for the remainder of their lifetime.

In summary, patients with connective tissue disorders comprise the greatest proportion of patients who will require modification or replacement of the aortic root in the setting of significant aortic valve insufficiency. Separate valve and graft replacement is the most expeditiously performed procedure and is most suitable for elderly patients or patients with poor ventricular function where peri-operative mortality, not long-term durability, is the primary concern. However, in younger patients, especially those with known or suspected connective tissue deficiency, root replacement is more appropriate. With a thorough understanding of the indications for aortic reconstruction, early referral for surgery can eliminate the risk of fatal aortic rupture or dissection. Valve-sparing techniques are still evolving and patient selection is of paramount importance in order to achieve acceptable intermediate and long-term results. Composite valve graft replacement remains the mainstay of surgical treatment for this disorder with exceptional reproducibility and durability. Operative risk can be close to zero in experienced centers and the long-term outcome is unmatched by any procedure to date.

References

1 Camacho MT, Cosgrove DM: Homografts in the treatment of prosthetic valve endocarditis. Semin Thorac Cardiovasc Surg 1995;7:32–37.

2 Bavaria JE, Pochettino A, Brinster DR, et al: New paradigms and improved results for the surgical treatment of acute type A dissection. Ann Surg 2001;234:336–343.

3 Girardi LN, Coselli JS: Inflammatory aneurysm of the ascending aorta and aortic arch. Ann Thorac Surg 1997;64:251–253.
4 Vaughan CJ, Casey IM, He J, et al: Identification of a chromosome 11q23.2–q24 locus for familial aortic aneurysm disease, a genetically heterogeneous disorder. Circulation 2001;103:2469–2475.
5 Elkins RC, Lane MM, McCue C, et al: Pulmonary autograft root replacement: Mid-term results. J Heart Valve Dis 1999;8:499–506.
6 Elkins RC, Lane MM: Autologous tissue in complex aortic valve disease. Semin Thorac Cardiovasc Surg 2001;13:267–272.
7 Pressler V, McNamara JJ: Thoracic aortic aneurysm: Natural history and treatment. J Thorac Cardiovasc Surg 1980;79:489–498.
8 Bickerstaff LK, Pairolero PC, Hollier LH, et al: Thoracic aortic aneurysms: A population-based study. Surgery 1986;92:1103–1108.
9 Perko MJ, Norgaard M, Herzog TM, et al: Unoperated aortic aneurysm: A survey of 170 patients. Ann Thorac Surg 1995;59:1204–1209.
10 Yun KL, Miller DC, Fann JI, et al: Composite valve graft versus separate aortic valve and ascending aortic replacement: Is there still a role for the separate procedure? Circulation 1997;96(suppl II):368–375.
11 Mora BN, Sundt TM, Ferrett R, et al: Bicuspid aortic valve disease and associated ascending aortic aneurysm: Composite root replacement or separate valve and graft replacement. Chest 1998;114:263S.
12 Yacoub M, Rasmi NRH, Sundt TM, et al: Fourteen-year experience with homovital homografts for aortic valve replacement. J Thorac Cardiovasc Surg 1995;110:186–194.
13 Kirklin JK, Smith D, Novick W, et al: Long-term function of cryopreserved aortic homografts: A ten-year study. J Thorac Cardiovasc Surg 1993;106:154–165.
14 David TE, Ivanov J, Armstrong S, et al: Late results of heart valve replacement with the Hancock II bioprosthesis. J Thorac Cardiovasc Surg 2001;121:268–278.
15 Yacoub MH, Fagan A, Stassano P, Radley-Smith R: Results of valve conserving operations for aortic regurgitation. Circulation 1983;68:311–321.
16 David TE: Aortic valve-sparing operations for aortic root aneurysm. Semin Thorac Cardiovasc Surg 2001;13:291–296.
17 David TE: Aortic valve-sparing operations: An update. Ann Thorac Surg 1999;67:1840–1842.
18 Yacoub MH, Gehle P, Chandrasekaran V, et al: Late results of a valve-preserving operation in patients with aneurysms of the ascending aorta and root. J Thorac Cardiovasc Surg 1998;115:1080–1090.
19 Bentall HH, DeBono A: A technique for complete replacement of the ascending aorta. Thorax 1968;23:338–339.
20 Girardi LN, Coselli JS: Aortic root replacement: Contemporary results utilizing the St Jude Medical/Hemashield composite valved conduit. Ann Thorac Surg 1997;64:1032–1038.
21 Kouchoukos NT, Wareing TH, Murphy SF, et al: Eleven-year experience with composite graft replacement of the ascending aorta and aortic valve. J Thorac Cardiovasc Surg 1986;92:691–705.
22 Gott VL, Greene PS, Alejo DE, et al: Replacement of the aortic root in patients with Marfan's syndrome. N Engl J Med 1999;340:1307.

Leonard N. Girardi, MD, Department of Cardiothoracic Surgery,
Weill Medical College of Cornell University, The New York-Presbyterian Hospital,
New York Weill Cornell Medical Center, 525 East 68th Street, New York, NY 10021 (USA)
Tel. +1 212 7465194, Fax +1 212 7468828, E-Mail lngirard@mail.med.cornell.edu

Borer JS, Isom OW (eds): Pathophysiology, Evaluation and Management of Valvular Heart Diseases.
Adv Cardiol. Basel, Karger, 2002, vol 39, pp 93–99

Technique and Results of the Modified Ross Procedure in Aortic Regurgitation versus Aortic Stenosis

Paul Stelzer

Beth Israel Medical Center, Division of Cardiac Surgery, New York, N.Y., USA

Fundamental to the Ross procedure (aortic valve replacement (AVR) with autologous pulmonary valve) is the concept of transferring the patient's normal, living, autologous pulmonary valve into the high pressure left side of the heart and putting the potentially troublesome replacement valve into the right side of the heart where the consequences of dysfunction are less severe and reoperation is easier. Donald Ross [1] first used the pulmonary autograft in 1967, implanting it the same way he did an aortic homograft 5 years earlier in the subcoronary 'freehand' technique.

The technical challenge of achieving a competent valve was addressed and improved by efforts to maintain the cylindrical geometry of the autograft placed within the native aorta [2, 3]. Diseased roots were completely replaced with homograft aortic valved conduits from the early 1970s [4]. Notably, these valves were consistently competent. This raised the question of doing the autograft as a full root replacement. There was significant concern that the delicate sinuses of the pulmonary artery might not allow safe reimplantation of the coronary ostia. In March 1987, the author did this modification for the first time and all of his subsequent autografts have been done as root replacements [5–7]. To clarify, this means a full, free-standing replacement of the aortic root with the pulmonary root. (It should be noted that Ross had actually done this very thing several times before that date when the aortic root was too diseased for his standard method.) Others soon adopted this as the technique of choice for this operation [8].

Patient Data

The author's personal experience includes 295 cases through April 2001. The age of these 228 men and 67 women ranged from 13 to 70 with a mean of 43.

Table 1. Concomitant procedures

	Patients, n[1]
Coronary artery bypass	35
Mitral valve procedures	30
Ascending aortic graft	9
Ascending aortorrhaphy	23
Closure of ASD	2
Closure of VSD	3
Septal myectomy	12
Closure of patent ductus	2
Total patients	98

[1] Some had multiple procedures.

Just under 10% of these patients had previous cardiac surgery (1 patient had three previous AVRs). Endocarditis (SBE) has been in the history of 35 patients; 12 were active (11 native, 1 bioprosthetic) at the time of surgery, and the other 23 were healed.

The primary pathology was aortic stenosis (AS) in 95, aortic regurgitation (AR) in 133, and mixed disease in the remaining 67. Approximately two thirds of mixed patients were predominant AS which splits the series almost equally between AR and AS. This forms the basis for comparing results between the two groups.

Additional procedures (often multiple) were performed in almost one third of patients (98 of the 295), most commonly coronary bypass and mitral valve (MV) repair (table 1). It is interesting to note that the additional procedures added an average of 17 min to the already long mean cross-clamp time of 146 min. The AS patient was more likely to have coronary bypass than was the AR. Mitral procedures (mostly rings) were more common in AR patients. Resection and graft replacement of the ascending aorta (n = 9) was more likely with AR and a lateral aortorrhaphy or aortoplasty (n = 23) more common with the post-stenotic dilatation seen with AS.

Results

There have been 6 operative deaths, 2% (table 2); 2 of the 3 bleeding deaths were in the active endocarditis setting leaving only 1 AS, 2 AR, and 1 mixed disease patient as mortalities. Clearly, there is no statistically significant difference here. Interestingly, coronary disease was involved in 3 of the deaths, so 5 of the

Table 2. Hospital mortality

Bleeding	3
Right ventricular failure	2
Resistant pneumonia	1
Total	6

Table 3. Morbidity (within 3 months)

Reoperation for bleeding	3
Heart block requiring pacemaker	2
Stroke	3[1]
TIA	1
Non-lethal RV dysfunction	3[2]
Temporary dialysis	2
Peri-operative myocardial infarction	1[3]
Deep sternal wound infection	1
Pulmonary embolus	1

[1] Lupus-, TTP- and PAF-related.
[2] Two required delayed primary sternal closure.
[3] Normal angiogram 6 months post-operatively.

6 deaths were in patients with either coronary disease or active endocarditis. Hospital mortality for patients with neither of these is therefore <0.5%. Three patients were discharged but died within the first 5 months after surgery (causes pulmonary embolus, ventricular tachycardia, and tamponade). These 3 bring the total early mortality up to 3%.

Morbidity has been low as well (table 3). Discharge on the fourth post-operative day is typical. Activity levels post-operatively have been virtually unrestricted with patients sky-diving, fighting fires, having children, and even doing ironman triathlons. Three months after he had his fourth aortic valve done as a Ross, 1 man reported running his first 9-min mile in 30 years.

On follow-up echo, no patient has developed stenosis of any significant degree – the flow patterns are normal because it is a normal human valve. There is moderate AR in <5% of patients. ‘Micro AR’ is commonly seen just as a ‘closing jet’ is seen with mechanical valves.

There was a right ventricular outflow tract (RVOT) gradient over 30 mm Hg in 6 patients. None has come to reoperation. There does appear to be an immune response to the homograft in the RVOT as evidenced by the development of panel-reactive antibody (PRA) positivity after homograft surgery. In a small

Table 4. Reoperations on the autograft

Endocarditis	2
Technical failure	5
Myxomatous disease progression	2
Total	9

percentage of patients reported to the International Ross Procedure Registry (1–2%) this is enough to produce severe scarring with significant obstruction of the pulmonary conduit distal to the valve. Percutaneous dilatation has been attempted with limited success and replacement with another cryopreserved homograft has produced a very rapid recurrence of the problem. Use of a totally decellularized homograft in this situation may prove successful as it evokes no antibody response.

Four patients have developed endocarditis in the post-operative, follow-up period. An IV drug user infected his pulmonary homograft twice, and 1 patient after a prostatic biopsy got mitral endocarditis. Both patients were cured with antibiotics alone. The 2 who developed SBE on the autograft both had active SBE at the original operation. These both required reoperation replacing the autografts with aortic homografts.

Reoperation has also been required for 7 others for a total of 9 autografts with significant AR – an incidence just under 3% (table 4). The 5 cases classified as technical failures were caused by inadequate support of the annulus or insufficient remodeling of the annulus so that it could accept the pulmonary valve without distortion. Of the 2 patients who developed myxomatous degeneration, 1 had AS and the other AR at original operation. This was intrinsic native tissue disease that could not be predicted. Six of the 9 had primary AR, but 2 of the 6 had endocarditis, so there is really no significant difference in incidence of reoperation between AS and AR patients.

Operations have been required on the MV in 5 patients, all for mitral regurgitation (MR). (Perhaps this is indicative of a weakness in the fibrous skeleton of the heart.) Three of these had double mechanical valve surgery for combined AR and MR. One developed bioprosthetic MR after Ross + MVR (itself after AVR/MVR). (After 12 years the porcine mitral required replacement and because there was a 30 mm Hg gradient across his pulmonary homograft this was replaced incidentally. The autograft valve was and is fine.) Of note, there has been no reoperative mortality. The living pulmonary root in the aortic position has proven very 'user friendly' for subsequent procedures.

Late mortality is listed in table 5. Clearly, some of this is not valve-related, but endocarditis is again a marker of poor outcome, accounting for 3 late deaths.

Table 5. Late mortality

Sudden death at 2 years, 7 years	2
Lung cancer at 7 months, 2 years	2
Seizure disorder at 20 months	1
Congestive failure at 30 months	1
Stroke at 8 years	1
Myocardial infarction at 8 years	1
Total late deaths	8

Discussion

How long will it last? The first one ever done was alive and well after 33 years. The RVOT reconstruction becomes the limiting factor. Data from Ross's group [3] shows 85% freedom from reoperation on the RVOT at 25 years. That is certainly better than survival of an aortic homograft in the aortic position, which has a 62% freedom from reoperation at 20 years according to Mark O'Brien's data in Australia.

The durability of the procedure is certainly dependent on the technical accuracy of the implantation. The author's data [7] and that of Elkins et al. [9] have demonstrated an advantage of the full root modification over the inclusion technique. It is just plain easier to get a reproducibly competent valve. The question remains as to whether the free-standing pulmonary root in the aortic position will dilate with continued years of systemic pressures [10]. We are still limited in our ability to detect incipient pathology of the native pulmonary valve but hopefully the human genome project will help us in this regard. One thing is sure: a dilated annulus and/or dilated distal aorta must be downsized and supported to prevent dilatation of the autograft root at either level, since such dilatation can render it incompetent over time. Dilatation of the sinuses alone looks frightening on echo and magnetic resonance scans, but may not cause regurgitation.

There are certain patients that should not have the Ross operation. Marfan's syndrome, a major connective tissue disorder, is a contraindication [11] (the fibrillin defect of the aortic wall affects the pulmonary as well). Active rheumatic disease may be a contraindication because it has attacked the autograft immediately after implantation, and certain other connective tissue diseases such as lupus may also attack the autograft. Some patients with bleeding disorders such as thrombocytopenia are a little more challenging, but they may also stand to benefit more by avoiding anticoagulation. Stopping platelet inhibitors pre-operatively and using aprotinin has proven very helpful. Valves diseased by endocarditis usually can be approached if the endocarditis is healed, but if there is real distortion at the root with an old abscess cavity, it may not be reconstructible. Active endocarditis can be approached if it is limited to the leaflets, but it is very difficult to do with a root abscess and in such a setting an aortic homograft is a great option [12].

Conclusions

The key differences between AS and AR and their impact on indications for the modified Ross procedure can be summarized as follows: the AR patient is more likely to have MR. The MR should be addressed first to make sure this is reparable before proceeding with the Ross. If the mitral cannot be repaired and both valves have rheumatic disease etiology, two mechanical valves work nicely. Rhythm is also an important consideration. Atrial fibrillation of long duration will usually require lifelong anticoagulation, so a mechanical valve is the logical choice.

Ventricular function is another key element. The patient with AR is more likely to have a dilated ventricle with limited systolic reserve. This requires meticulous attention to myocardial protection. The corollary is: 'Don't wait forever to send the asymptomatic young patient with AR to surgery.' The AS ventricle certainly tolerates the operation better, even though it takes a little longer to excise the valve. The coronaries ought to be good, or ought to have something relatively simple to fix, preferably with arterial conduit.

As for the root itself, its size and its elasticity are usually both less in patients with AS, so support is not required. The opposite is true for AR and support should almost always be used, often on both ends. Incorporation of a measured strip of Teflon felt works very nicely to downsize and fix either the annulus or the sinotubular junction to prevent stretching. The patient with AR is also slightly more likely to have had a history of endocarditis, so careful consideration must be given to the root architecture in order to determine that it can be properly reconstructed. It is important to remember that the pulmonary root is a totally unsupported device and it is going to assume the shape of what it is put into unless that shape is modified. This is a particularly serious problem in the setting of active or healed root abscess.

Excess ascending aorta must also be addressed. As previously stated, true ascending aneurysm is more likely with AR than with AS. Post-stenotic dilatation can usually be wedged out and sewn up primarily. True aneurysms should be resected and replaced with a graft. Furthermore, in cases where the root itself is aneurysmal or there is sinus of Valsalva aneurysm, it may be wise to place a 'jacket' of graft material completely around the autograft. With these special considerations, the operation can be extended to complex situations in young patients who would otherwise just get a mechanical valved conduit.

The older the patient, the less these indications should be stretched. Age is not so important as life expectancy and that should be at least 25 years. Other easier alternatives become increasingly attractive in older patients. Ideal patients are <45, but it is very reasonable to offer the Ross to people up to age 65 if other factors are favorable.

In conclusion, the full root modification of Ross's pulmonary autograft can be done with an acceptably low mortality and morbidity and offers long-term durability without anticoagulation [7, 13, 14]. This holds true for properly selected patients with most aortic valve disease, whether it be primarily AR, AS, or a mixed lesion. The risk and durability are influenced by the patient's age, the presence of active infection and concomitant coronary artery disease.

References

1 Ross DN: Replacement of aortic and mitral valves with a pulmonary autograft. Lancet 1967;ii: 956–958.
2 Stelzer P: Pulmonary autograft replacement of the aortic valve; in Emery RW, Arom KV (eds): The Aortic Valve. Philadelphia, Hanley & Belfus, 1991, pp 227–234.
3 Chambers JC, Sommerville J, Stone S, Ross DN: Pulmonary autograft procedure for aortic valve disease. Long-term results of the pioneer series. Circulation 1997;96:2206–2214.
4 Stelzer P, Elkins RC: Homograft valves and conduits: Applications in cardiac surgery. Curr Probl Surg 1989;26:381–452.
5 Stelzer P, Elkins RC: Pulmonary autograft: An American experience. J Cardiac Surg 1987;2: 429–433.
6 Stelzer P, Jones DJ, Elkins RC: Aortic root replacement using pulmonary autograft. Circulation 1989;80(suppl III):209–213.
7 Stelzer P, Weinrauch S, Tranbaugh RF: Ten years' experience with the modified Ross procedure. J Thorac Cardiovasc Surg 1998;115:1091–1100.
8 Kouchoukos NT, Davila-Roman VG, Spray TL, Murphy SF, Perrilo JB: Replacement of the aortic root with a pulmonary autograft in children and young adults with aortic valve disease. N Engl J Med 1994;330:1–6.
9 Elkins RC, Lane MM, McCue C: Pulmonary autograft reoperation; incidence and management. Ann Thorac Surg 1996;62:450–455.
10 David TE, Omran A, Webb G, Rakowski H, Armstrong S, Sun Z: Geometric mismatch of the aortic and pulmonary roots causes aortic insufficiency after the Ross procedure. J Thorac Cardiovasc Surg 1996;112:1231–1239.
11 Oury JH: Clinical aspects of the Ross procedure: Indications and contraindications. Semin Cardiovasc Surg 1996;4:328–335.
12 Oswalt J: Management of aortic infective endocarditis by autograft valve replacement. J Heart Valve Dis 1994;3:377–379.
13 Doty DB: Aortic valve replacement with homograft and autograft. Semin Thorac Cardiovasc Surg 1996;8:249–258.
14 Dossche KM, de la Riviere AB, Morshuis SJ, Schepens MAAM, Ernst SM, van den Brand JJ: Aortic root replacement with the pulmonary autograft: An invariably competent aortic valve? Ann Thorac Surg 1999;68:1302–1307.

Paul Stelzer, MD, Beth Israel Medical Center, Division of Cardiac Surgery,
1st Avenue at 16th Street, New York, NY 10003 (USA)

Borer JS, Isom OW (eds): Pathophysiology, Evaluation and Management of Valvular Heart Diseases.
Adv Cardiol. Basel, Karger, 2002, vol 39, pp 100–113

Percutaneous Mitral Balloon Valvuloplasty. Does It Really Last as Long and Do as Well as Surgery?

Igor F. Palacios

Cardiac Unit, Department of Medicine, Massachusetts General Hospital,
Harvard Medical School, Boston, Mass., USA

Surgical mitral commissurotomy has been demonstrated to be useful in the treatment of patients with symptomatic mitral stenosis (MS) [1–6]. Both open and closed mitral commissurotomy have resulted in excellent immediate and long-term improvement. Since its introduction in 1984 [7], percutaneous mitral balloon valvuloplasty (PMV) has been demonstrated to be effective for treatment of patients with MS [8–16]. As a result, today PMV is an alternative treatment for patients with symptomatic MS. In addition, considerable data on the immediate and long-term results of PMV have been recently accumulated. These data include results from PMV series and from some randomized trials of surgical commissurotomy vs. PMV [8–19].

The Massachusetts General Hospital Experience

Patient Population. The patient population included 879 consecutive patients who underwent 939 PMV between July 1986 and July 2000 (table 1). There were 160 males and 719 females with a mean age of 55 ± 15 years. Atrial fibrillation was present in 430 (49%) patients, 143 patients had a history of previous surgical mitral commissurotomy and presented with MS. Mitral regurgitation (MR) ⩾ grade 2 by the Sellers' classification, was present in 66 (7%) patients and significant mitral valve (MV) calcification under fluoroscopy (⩾2+) was present in 230 (26.4%). Most patients were severely limited by congestive heart failure with 655 (74.5%) in New York Heart Association (NYHA) functional classes III and IV.

Six hundred and ninety-five PMV procedures were performed using the double balloon technique, 237 with the Inoue technique and 7 with a combination of both techniques as previously described [8, 20, 21]. Right and left heart

Table 1. Baseline characteristics

Number of patients	879 (939 PMV)
Age, years	55 ± 15
Female gender	719 (82%)
Atrial fibrillation	430 (49%)
Previous commissurotomy	143 (16%)
Mitral regurgitation $\geqslant 2+$	57 (6.5%)
Fluoroscopic calcium $\geqslant 2+$	230 (26%)
NYHA class	
Class I	12 (2%)
Class II	212 (24%)
Class III	539 (61%)
Class IV	116 (13%)

pressure measurements, cardiac outputs and oxygen saturations were assessed before and after PMV. The MV area (MVA) was calculated using the Gorlin formula [22]. Left ventriculography was performed before and after PMV to assess the severity of MR using the Sellers' classification [23].

Selection of Patients. The criteria for patients to be considered for PMV include (1) symptomatic MS, (2) no recent embolic event, (3) <2+ MR by the Sellers' classification, (4) no evidence of left atrial thrombus on two-dimensional (2D)-echocardiography and transesophageal echocardiography. Patients in atrial fibrillation and patients with previous embolic episodes are required to be anticoagulated with warfarin and to have a therapeutic prothrombin time for at least 3 months before PMV.

Technique of PMV. There is not a unique technique of PMV. Most of the PMV techniques require transseptal left heart catheterization and use of the antegrade approach. Antegrade PMV can be accomplished using either the Inoue balloon or the double balloon technique [8, 20, 21]. Recently, a technique of PMV using a newly designed metallic valvulotome was introduced [24]. The device consists of a detachable metallic cylinder with two articulated bars screwed onto the distal end of a disposable catheter whose proximal end is connected to activating pliers. Squeezing the pliers opens the bars up to a maximum of 40 mm. The results with this device are at least comparable to those of the other balloon techniques of PMV. However, multiple uses after sterilization should markedly decrease procedural costs.

Immediate Results. The hemodynamic findings before and after PMV of the overall patient population are shown in figure 1 and table 2. Procedure success was defined as a post-PMV MVA $\geqslant 1.5\,cm^2$ and post-PMV MR <3+ according with Sellers' class. PMV resulted in an increase in MVA from 0.9 ± 0.3 to $1.9 \pm 0.7\,cm^2$ ($p < 0.0001$). There is an inverse relationship between echo score (Echo-Sc), and both post-PMV MVA and PMV success

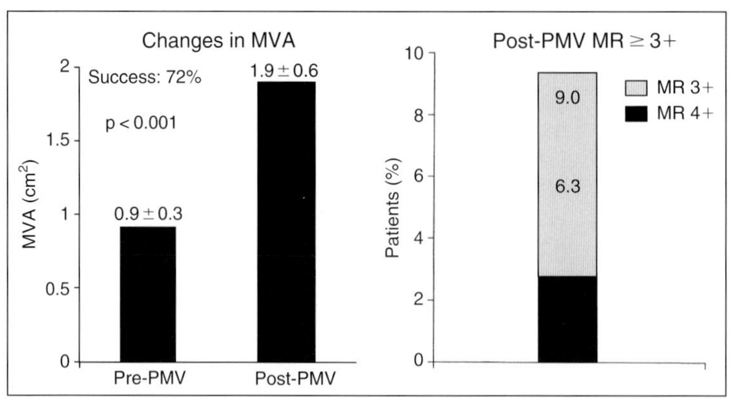

Fig. 1. Changes in MVA produced by PMV (right) and frequency of 3+ and 4+ post-PMV MR (left) for the overall population. MVA = Mitral valve area, MR = mitral regurgitation, PMV = percutaneous mitral balloon valvuloplasty.

Table 2. Hemodynamic changes produced by PMV

	Pre-PMV	Post-PMV	p value
Mitral valve area	0.9 ± 0.3	1.9 ± 0.7	< 0.0001
Mitral gradient	14 ± 6	6 ± 3	< 0.0001
Cardiac output	3.9 ± 1.1	4.5 ± 1.3	< 0.0001
Mean PA	36 ± 13	29 ± 11	< 0.0001
Mean LA	25 ± 7	17 ± 7	< 0.0001
EBDA/BSA	3.62 ± 0.49 cm^2/m^2		
PMV success	72%		
Post-PMV MR 3+	56 (6.0%)		
Post-PMV MR 4+	32 (3.4%)		
QP/QS > 1.5 : 1	50 (5.3%)		

EBDA = Effective balloon dilating area; BSA = body surface area; MR = mitral regurgitation; PMV = percutaneous mitral balloon valvuloplasty; QP/QS = pulmonary to systemic flow ratio.

(fig. 2). Patients with Echo-Sc ≤8 had larger increase in post-PMV MVA (2.0 ± 0.6 cm^2 vs. 1.6 ± 0.6 cm^2; $p < 0.0001$). Procedural success was 71.7% for the overall group, with patients with Echo-Sc ≤8 having a higher procedural success (79.0 vs. 56.4%; $p < 0.0001$). Two hundred and sixty-six patients had unsuccessful procedures because of a post-PMV MVA <1.5 cm^2 (178 patients) and post-PMV MR ≥3 Sellers' grade (88 patients). Although a suboptimal result

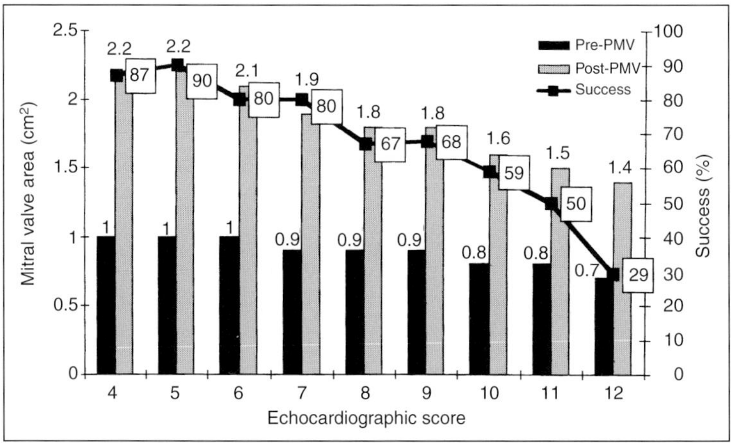

Fig. 2. Relationship between the echocardiographic score and PMV success.

occurred in 21% of the patients, a post-PMV MVA $\leq$1.0 cm^2 (critical MVA) was present in only 7% of these patients.

Multiple stepwise logistic regression analysis identified larger pre-PMV MVA, less degree of pre-PMV MR, younger age, absence of previous surgical commissurotomy, male sex and Echo-Sc $\leq$8 as independent predictors of procedural success. As shown in table 3, our results are similar to those of other large PMV series previously published.

In-Hospital Adverse Events. The incidence of major adverse in-hospital events is shown in table 4. There were 18 (1.9%) in-hospital deaths, and 6 (0.6%) of them were procedure-related deaths. Severe post-PMV MR ($\geq$3 Sellers' grade) occurred in 9.4% of the patients, with Sellers' grade III in 6%, and Sellers' grade IV in 3.4%. In-hospital MV replacement (MVR) was performed in 3.3% of the patients with a higher incidence in patients with Echo-Sc >8. Emergent MVR was required in 1.4% of the patients. Other complications included 1% incidence of pericardial tamponade, 5.3% of left to right shunt with a pulmonary to systemic flow ratio >1.5 : 1, 1.8% of thromboembolic events and 0.5% of complete atrioventricular block. As shown in table 4, our results are similar to those of other large PMV series.

Clinical Follow-Up. Clinical follow-up information was available in 844 (96%) of the overall patient population at a mean follow-up time of 4.2 ± 3.7 years. For the entire population, there were 110 deaths (25 noncardiac), 234 MVR and 54 redo PMV accounting for a total of 398 patients (47%) with combined events (death, MVR or redo PMV). Of the remaining 446 patients that were free of combined events, 418 (94%) were in NYHA class I or II.

Table 3. Changes in mitral valve area

Author	Institution	Patients, n	Age	Pre-PMV (cm^2)	Post-PMV (cm^2)
Palacios	MGH	860	57 ± 12	0.9 ± 0.3	2.0 ± 0.2
Vahanian [38]	Tenon	1,514	45 ± 15	1.0 ± 0.2	1.9 ± 0.3
Stefanadis [39]	Athens Univ.	438	44 ± 11	1.0 ± 0.3	2.1 ± 0.5
Chen [40]	Guangzhou	4,832	37 ± 12	1.1 ± 0.3	2.1 ± 0.2
NHLBI [41, 42]	Multicenter	738	54 ± 12	1.0 ± 0.4	2.0 ± 0.2
Inoue	Takeda	527	50 ± 10	1.1 ± 0.1	2.0 ± 0.1
Inoue Registry	Multicenter	1,251	53 ± 15	1.0 ± 0.3	1.8 ± 0.6
Farhat [43]	Fattouma	463	33 ± 12	1.0 ± 0.2	2.2 ± 0.4
Arora [44]	G.B. Pan	600	27 ± 8	0.8 ± 0.2	2.2 ± 0.4
Cribier [45]	Ruen	153	36 ± 15	1.0 ± 0.2	2.2 ± 0.4

Table 4. Complications of PMV

Author	Patients, n	Mortality (%)	Tamponade (%)	Severe MR (%)	Embolism (%)
Palacios	860	0.3	0.6	3.3	1.0
Vahanian [38]	1,514	0.4	0.3	3.4	0.3
Stefanadis [39]	438	0.2	0.0	3.4	0.0
Chen [40]	4,832	0.1	0.8	1.4	0.5
NHLBI [41, 42]	738	3.0	4.0	3.0	3.0
Inoue	527	0.0	1.6	1.9	0.6
Inoue Registry	1,251	0.6	1.4	3.8	0.9
Farhat [43]	463	0.4	0.7	4.6	2.0
Arora [44]	600	1.0	1.3	1.0	0.5
Cribier [45]	153	0.0	0.7	1.4	0.7

Endpoint events occurred less frequently in the 575 patients with Echo-Sc ≤8 than in those with Echo-Sc >8.

As shown in figures 3 and 4, actuarial survival and event-free survival rates throughout the follow-up period were significantly better in patients with Echo-Sc ≤8 (12-year survival = 82% for patients with Echo-Sc ≤8 vs. 57% for patients with Echo-Sc >8; $p < 0.001$). Event-free survival (38 vs. 22%; $p < 0.0001$) at 12 years' follow-up were also significantly higher for patients with Echo-Sc ≤8. Survival rates were 82 and 56%, respectively, when only patients with successful PMV were included in the analysis. Event-free survival rates were 41 and 23%, respectively, when only patients with successful PMV were included in the analysis.

Cox regression analysis identified post-PMV MR ≥3+, Echo-Sc >8, age, prior commissurotomy, NYHA functional class IV, pre-PMV MR ≥2+ and

3 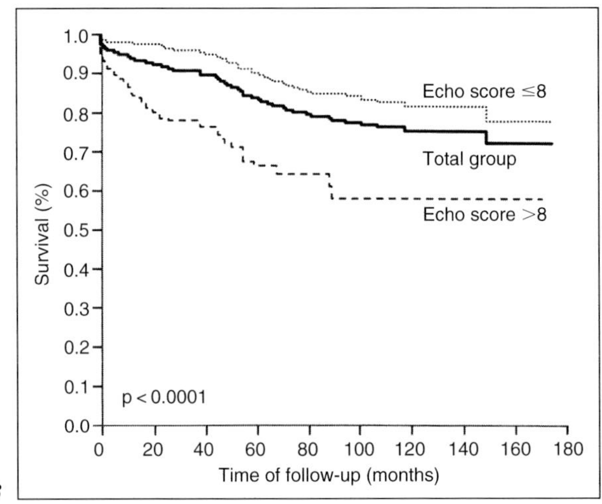

4 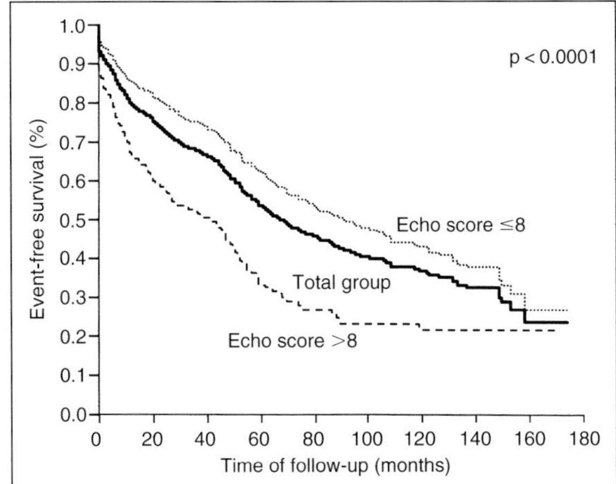

Fig. 3. Kaplan-Meier survival estimates for patients with echocardiographic scores ⩽8 and >8 [modified from Palacios IF et al: Which patients benefit from percutaneous mitral balloon valvuloplasty? Circulation 2002;105, with permission].

Fig. 4. Kaplan-Meier event-free survival estimates (alive and free of MVR or redo PMV) for patients with Echo-Sc ⩽8 and >8 [modified from Palacios IF et al: Which patients benefit from percutaneous mitral balloon valvuloplasty? Circulation 2002;105, with permission].

post-PMV pulmonary artery pressure as independent predictors of combined events at long-term follow-up.

The Echocardiographic Score. Patient selection is fundamental in predicting immediate outcome and follow-up results of PMV and surgical commissurotomy procedures. In addition to clinical examination, echocardiographic evaluation of the MV and fluoroscopic screening for valvular calcification are the most important steps in patient selection for successful outcome. The evaluation of candidates for PMV requires a precise evaluation of both valve morphology and function for preprocedure decision-making and follow-up of the patients. 2D-echocardiography is currently the most widely used noninvasive technique for the evaluation of the morphologic characteristics of the MV, subvalvular apparatus and the valve annular size. An important predictor of the immediate and long-term results of PMV is a morphologic echocardiographic score developed at the Massachusetts General Hospital [25, 26]. In this score each of the following – leaflet mobility, leaflet thickening, valvular calcification and subvalvular disease – are scored from 1+ to 4+, yielding a maximum total echocardiographic score of 16. A higher score would represent a heavily calcified, thickened and immobile valve with extensive thickening and calcification of the subvalvular apparatus. Among the four components of the echocardiographic score, valve leaflets thickening and subvalvular disease correlate the best with the increase in MVA produced by PMV. An inverse relationship between the immediate and long-term results produced by PMV and the echo cardiographic score has been demonstrated [11, 12, 15]. Patients with lower echocardiographic scores have a higher likelihood of having a good outcome from PMV with minimal complications and a hemodynamic and clinical improvement that persist at long-term follow-up.

Other Predictors of PMV Outcome. The reliability of the echocardiographic score for predicting results of PMV is not optimal because result of the PMV is related to other factors such as the presence of fluoroscopic MV calcification, the age and gender of the patient, the presence of atrial fibrillation, pre-PMV MR and pulmonary hypertension, a history of previous surgical commissurotomy, the technique of PMV (double balloon vs. Inoue), the severity of MS before PMV and the effective balloon dilating area [8–11].

As shown in figures 5 and 6, age is an important factor for determining the immediate and long-term outcome of PMV [8–11, 27]. We have previously reported a 46% success rate in patients ⩾65 years. In this population, independent predictors of success included a lower echocardiographic score, lower pre-PMV NYHA functional class and a larger pre-PMV MVA. A low echocardiographic score was the strongest independent predictor of survival, and the lack of MV calcification was the strongest predictor of event-free survival [27].

The presence of fluoroscopically visible calcification on the MV is another important factor that influences the success of PMV [28]. Patients with heavily calcified MV have a poorer immediate outcome as reflected in a smaller post-PMV MVA. The long-term survival and event-free survival are significantly lower for patients with calcified MV than for those with uncalcified valves. Furthermore, the survival and event-free survival curves become worse

5 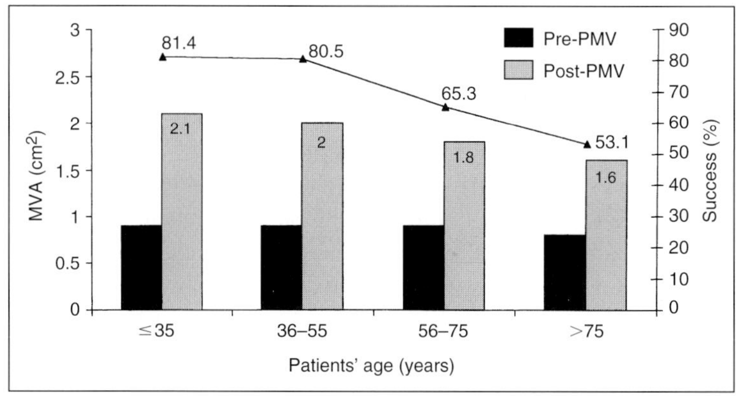

6 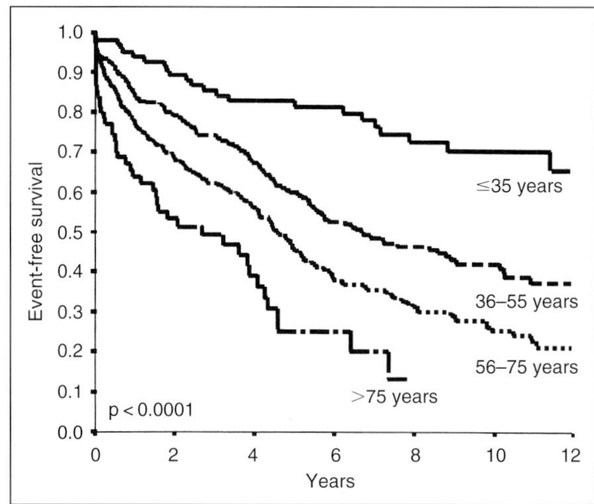

Fig. 5. Relationship between patients' age and changes in MVA after PMV, and relationship between patients' age and PMV success.

Fig. 6. Kaplan-Meier event-free survival estimates (alive and free of MVR or redo PMV) for patients ≤35, 36–55, 56–75 and >75 years old.

as the severity of valvular calcification becomes more severe. These findings are in agreement with several follow-up studies of surgical commissurotomy, which demonstrated that patients with calcified MV had a significantly poorer survival compared to those patients with uncalcified valves.

The presence of atrial fibrillation is adversely related to the outcome of PMV. Patients in atrial fibrillation have clinical and morphologic characteristics associated with inferior results after PMV such as older age, higher prevalence of echocardiographic scores >8 and history of previous surgical commissurotomy.

In patients with atrial fibrillation, PMV resulted in inferior immediate and long-term outcomes as reflected in a smaller post-PMV MVA and a lower event-free survival at a long-term follow-up. In patients with atrial fibrillation post-PMV MR ⩾grade 3, echocardiographic score >8 and pre-PMV NYHA class IV are independent predictors of combined events at follow-up [29].

PMV also has been safe in patients with previous surgical mitral commissurotomy [30, 31]. Although a good immediate outcome is frequently achieved in these patients, event-free survival is greater among those patients without previous commissurotomy. However, when patients are carefully selected using an echocardiographic score ⩽8, the immediate outcome and long-term follow-up results are excellent and similar to those seen in patients without a history of previous surgical commissurotomy [31].

The degree of pulmonary artery hypertension before PMV is inversely related to the immediate and long-term outcome of PMV. Chen et al. [32] divided 564 patients undergoing PMV at the Massachusetts General Hospital into three groups on the basis of the pulmonary vascular resistance (PVR) obtained at cardiac catheterization immediately prior to PMV: group I with a PVR ⩽250 $dyn \cdot s/cm^{-5}$ (normal/mildly elevated resistance) comprised 332 patients (59%); group II with a PVR between 251 and 400 $dyn \cdot s/cm^{-5}$ (moderately elevated resistance) comprised 110 patients (19.5%), and group III with a PVR ⩾400$dyn \cdot s/cm^{-5}$ comprised 122 patients (21.5%). Patients in groups I and II were younger, had less severe heart failure symptoms measured by NYHA class and a lower prevalence of echocardiographic scores >8, atrial fibrillation and calcium noted on fluoroscopy than patients in group III. Before and after PMV, patients with higher PVR had a smaller MVA, lower cardiac output, and higher mean pulmonary artery pressure. For group I, II and III patients, the immediate success rates for PMV were 68, 56 and 45%, respectively. Therefore, patients in the group with severely elevated pulmonary artery resistance before the procedure had lower immediate success rates of PMV. At long-term follow-up patients with severely elevated PVRs had a significantly lower survival and event-free survival (survival with freedom from MV surgery or NYHA class III or IV heart failure).

The degree of tricuspid regurgitation (TR) before PMV is inversely related to the immediate and long-term outcome of PMV. Sagie et al. [33] divided patients undergoing PMV at the Massachusetts General Hospital into three groups on the basis of the degree of TR determined by 2D and color flow Doppler echocardiography before PMV. Patients with severe TR before PMV were older, had more severe heart failure measured by NYHA class and a higher prevalence of echocardiographic scores >8, atrial fibrillation and calcified MV on fluoroscopy than patients with mild or moderate TR. Patients with severe TR had smaller MVA before and after PMV than patients with mild or moderate TR.

At long-term follow-up, patients with severe TR had a significantly lower survival and event-free survival.

In patients identified as optimal candidates for PMV, this technique results in excellent immediate and long-term outcome. Optimal candidates for PMV are those patients meeting the following characteristics: (a) age <55 years old, (b) normal sinus rhythm, (c) echocardiographic score ≤8, (d) no fluoroscopic MV calcification, and (e) pre-PMV MR ≤1+ Seller's grade. From 780 consecutive patients undergoing PMV, we identified 202 patients with optimal pre-procedure characteristics. In these patients, PMV resulted in an 81% success rate and a 3.4% incidence of major in-hospital combined events (death and/or MVR). In these patients, PMV resulted in a 97% survival and 76% event-free survival at a median follow-up of 61 months [34].

Comparison of PMV with Surgical MV Commissurotomy

Comparison between PMV and surgical commissurotomy techniques is difficult in view of differences in clinical and MV morphology characteristics among different series. Most surgical series have involved a younger population with optimal MV morphology, i.e., pliable with no calcification and no evidence of subvalvular disease. Differences in age and valve morphology may account for the lower survival and event-free survival of PMV series from the USA and Europe. For example in the series from the Massachusetts General Hospital, 497 patients with echocardiographic scores ≤8 and a mean age of 51 ± 14 years have a 85% survival and 45% event-free survival at 8-year follow-up. In contrast, 237 patients with echocardiographic scores >8 and a mean age of 63 ± 14 years have a 55% 8-year survival with only 20% freedom from combined events.

A larger number of patients with higher echocardiographic scores and MV calcification may account for the 5-year 76% survival and a 51% combined event-free survival reported by Cohen et al. [12] in a group of 146 patients undergoing PMV. Furthermore, 39% of the patients in this later series were considered to be high surgical risk candidates due to the presence of important coexisting conditions or advanced age. On the contrary, survival and event-free survival after PMV in optimal patients for this technique appear to be similar to those reported after surgical mitral commissurotomy, as suggested from the previously noted series from the Massachusetts General Hospital in 202 optimal candidates.

In patients with optimal MV morphology, surgical mitral commissurotomy has favorable long-term hemodynamic and symptomatic improvement. Similarly to PMV, patients with advanced age, calcified MV, and those with atrial fibrillation had a poorer survival and event-free survival. Several studies have compared the immediate and follow-up results of PMV vs. surgical commissurotomy in optimal patients for these techniques. The results of these studies have been controversial showing either superior outcome from PMV [35, 36] or no significant differences between both techniques [17, 18, 36]. Patel et al. [35] randomized 45 patients with MS and optimal MV morphology to closed surgical commissurotomy and to PMV [35]. He demonstrated a larger increase in MVA with PMV ($2.1 \pm 0.7\,cm^2$ vs. $1.3 \pm 0.3\,cm^2$). Shrivastava et al. [36] compared the results of single balloon PMV, double balloon PMV and closed surgical commissurotomy in three groups of 20 patients each. The MVA post-intervention was larger for the double balloon technique of PMV. Post-intervention valve areas were $1.9 \pm 0.8\,cm^2$, $1.5 \pm 0.4\,cm^2$ and $1.5 \pm 0.5\,cm^2$ for the double balloon, single balloon and closed surgical commissurotomy techniques respectively. On the other hand, Arora et al. [37] randomized 200 patients with a mean age of 19 ± 7 years and MS with optimal MV morphology to PMV and to closed mitral commissurotomy. Both procedures resulted in similar post-intervention MVAs ($2.39 \pm 0.9\,cm^2$ vs. $2.2 \pm 0.9\,cm^2$ for the PMV and the mitral commissurotomy groups respectively) and no significant differences in event-free survival at a mean follow-up period of 22 ± 6 months. Restenosis documented by echocardiography was low in both groups, 5% in the PMV group and 4% in the closed commissurotomy group.

Although these initial randomized trials results of PMV vs. surgical commissurotomy are encouraging and favor PMV for the treatment of patients with rheumatic MS with suitable MV anatomy, there was a need for long-term follow-up studies to define more precisely the role of PMV in these patients. Turi et al. [17] randomized 40 patients with severe MS to PMV and to closed surgical commissurotomy. The post-intervention MVA ($1.6 \pm 0.6\,cm^2$ vs. $1.6 \pm 0.7\,cm^2$) and 10-year follow-up were similar in both groups. Reyes et al. [18] randomized 60 patients with severe MS and favorable valvular anatomy to PMV and to surgical commissurotomy. They reported no significant differences in immediate outcome, complications and 7-year follow-up between both groups of patients. Improvement was maintained in both groups, but MVA at follow-up were larger in the PMV group ($2.4 \pm 0.6\,cm^2$ vs. $1.8 \pm 0.4\,cm^2$).

In a cohort of patients with optimal MV anatomy, Farhat et al. [19] reported similar immediate and long-term results of PMV to those obtained with open surgical commissurotomy and significantly superior to those obtained with closed surgical commissurotomy. The post-intervention MVA achieved with PMV were similar to the one obtained after open surgical commissurotomy ($2.5 \pm 0.5\,cm^2$ vs. $2.2 \pm 0.4\,cm^2$) but larger than those obtained after closed commissurotomy. These initial changes resulted in an excellent long-term follow-up in the group of patients treated with PMV, which was comparable with the open commissurotomy group and superior to the closed commissurotomy group. The inferior results of closed mitral commissurotomy presented by Farhat et al. [19] are in disagreement with previous studies showing no significant differences in immediate

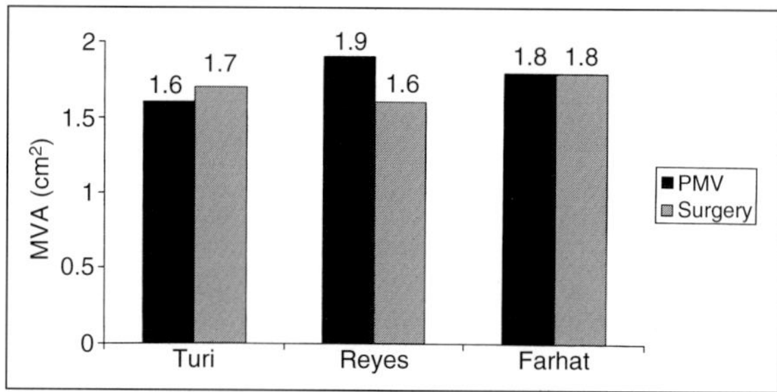

Fig. 7. Seven-year follow-up mitral valve areas of randomized studies of PMV vs. closed (Turi) and open surgical commissurotomy (Reyes, Farhat).

and follow-up results between PMV and closed surgical mitral commissurotomy [18, 37]. However, the increase in MVA after closed commissurotomy is not uniform and often is unsatisfactory. Regardless of this controversy, the long-term follow-up results of the studies of Turi, Reyes and Farhat provide further support to the conclusion that PMV should be the procedure of choice for treatment of patients with rheumatic MS (fig. 7).

Conclusions

PMV results in excellent hemodynamic and clinical improvement in the majority of patients with MS. In hospital complications, immediate and long-term results are similar to those of surgical commissurotomy. Since open commissurotomy is associated with a thoracotomy, need for cardiopulmonary bypass, higher cost, longer length of hospital stay and a longer period of convalescence, PMV should be the procedure of choice for the treatment of patients with rheumatic MS who are optimal candidates for PMV from the clinical and morphological point of view.

References

1 Harken DE, Ellis LB, Ware PF, Norman LR: The surgical treatment of mistral stenosis. I. Valvuloplasty. N Engl J Med 1948;239:801–809.

2 Harken DE, Dexter L, Ellis LB, Farrand RE, Dickson JF: The surgery of mitral stenosis. III. Finger fracture valvuloplasty. Ann Surg 1951;134:722–742.

3 Ellis LB, Harken DE, Black H: A clinical study of 1,000 consecutive cases of mitral stenosis two to nine years after mitral valvuloplasty. Circulation 1959;19:803–820.

4 Ellis LB, Singh JB, Morales DD, Harken DE: Fifteen to twenty years' study of one thousand patients undergoing closed mitral valvuloplasty. Circulation 1973;48:357–364.

5 Hoeksema TD, Wallace RB, Kirkling JW: Closed mitral commissurotomy. Am J Cardiol 1966;17:825–828.

6 Nathaniels EK, Moncure AC, Scanell JG: A fifteen-year follow-up study of closed mitral valvuloplasty. Ann Thorac Surg 1970;10:27–36.
7 Inoue K, Owaki T, Nakamura T, Kitamura F, Miyamoto N: Clinical application of transvenous mitral commissurotomy by a new balloon catheter. J Thorac Cardiovasc Surg 1984;87:394–402.
8 Palacios IF, Block PC, Brandi S, Blanco P, Casal H, Pulido JI, Munoz S, D'Empaire G, Ortega MA, Jacobs M, Vlahakes G: Percutaneous balloon valvotomy for patients with severe mitral stenosis. Circulation 1987;75:778–784.
9 Iung BL, Garbarz E, Michaud P, et al: Late results of percutaneous mitral commissurotomy in a series of 1,024 patients. Analysis of late clinical deterioration: Frequency, anatomic findings and predictive factors. Circulation 1999;99:3272–3278.
10 Hernandez R, Banuelos C, Alfonso F, et al: Long-term clinical and echocardiographic follow-up after percutaneous mitral valvuloplasty with the Inoue balloon. Circulation 1999;99:1580–1586.
11 Palacios IF, Block PC, Wilkins GT, Weyman AE: Follow-up of patients undergoing mitral balloon valvotomy: Analysis of factors determining restenosis. Circulation 1989;79:573–579.
12 Cohen DJ, Kuntz RE, Gordon SPF, et al: Predictors of long-term outcome after percutaneous mitral valvuloplasty. N Engl J Med 1991;327:1329–1335.
13 Hung JS, Chern MS, Wu JJ, et al: Short- and long-term results of catheter balloon percutaneous transvenous mitral commissurotomy. Am J Cardiol 1991;67:854–862.
14 Palacios IF: Farewell to surgical mitral commissurotomy for many patients. Circulation 1998;97: 223–226.
15 Dean LS, Mickel M, Bonan R, et al: Four-year follow-up of patients undergoing percutaneous balloon mitral commissurotomy. A report from the National Heart, Lung and Blood Institute Balloon Valvuloplasty Registry. J Am Coll Cardiol 1996;28:1452–1457.
16 Stefanides C, Stratos C, Pitsavos C, et al: Retrograde nontransseptal balloon mitral valvuloplasty. Immediate results and long-term follow-up. Circulation 1992;85:1760–1767.
17 Turi ZG, Reyes VP, Raju BS, et al: Percutaneous balloon versus surgical closed commissurotomy for mitral stenosis: A prospective, randomized trial. Circulation 1991;83:1179–1185.
18 Reyes VP, Raju BS, Wynne J, et al: Percutaneous balloon valvuloplasty compared with open surgical commissurotomy for mitral stenosis. N Engl J Med 1994;331:961–967.
19 Farhat MB, Ayari M, Maatouk F, et al: Percutaneous balloon versus surgical closed and open mitral commissurotomy: Seven-year follow-up results of a randomized trial. Circulation 1998;97: 245–250.
20 Feldman T, Herrmann HC, Inoue K: Technique of percutaneous transvenous mitral commissurotomy using the Inoue balloon catheter. Cathet Cardiovasc Diagn 1994(suppl 2):26–34.
21 Lau KW, Gao W, Ding ZP, Hung JS: Immediate and long-term results of percutaneous Inoue balloon mitral commissurotomy with use of a simple height-derived balloon sizing method for the stepwise dilation technique. Mayo Clinic Proc 1996;71:556–663.
22 Gorlin R, Gorlin SG: Hydraulic formula for calculation of the area of the stenotic mitral valve, other cardiac valves and central circulatory shunts. Am Heart J 1951;41:1–29.
23 Sellers RD, Levy MJ, Amplatz K, Lillehei CW: Left retrograde cardioangiography in acquired cardiac disease. Am J Cardiol 1964;14:437–447.
24 Cribier A, Eltchaninoff H, Koning R, Rath PC, Arora R, Imam A, El-Sayed M, Dani S, Derumeaux G, Benichou J, Tron C, Janorkar S, Pontier G, Letac B: Percutaneous mechanical mitral commissurotomy with a newly designed metallic valvulotome. Circulation 1999;99:793–799.
25 Wilkins GT, Weyman AE, Abascal VM, Block PC, Palacios IF: Percutaneous mitral valvotomy: An analysis of echocardiographic variables related to outcome and the mechanism of dilatation. Br Heart J 1988;60:299-308.
26 Abascal VM, Wilkins GT, Choong CY, Palacios IF, Block PC, Weyman AE: Echocardiographic evaluation of mitral valve structure and function in patients followed for at least 6 months after percutaneous balloon mitral valvuloplasty. J Am Coll Cardiol 1988;12:606–615.
27 Tuzcu EM, Block PC, Griffin BP, Newell JB, Palacios IF: Immediate and long-term outcome of percutaneous mitral valvotomy in patients 65 years and older. Circulation 1992;85:963–971.
28 Tuzcu EM, Block PC, Griffin B, Dinsmore R, Newell JB, Palacios IF: Percutaneous mitral balloon valvotomy in patients with calcific mitral stenosis: Immediate and long-term outcome. J Am Coll Cardiol 1994;23:1604–1609.

29 Leon M, Harrell L, Mahdi N, Simosa H, Pathan A, Lopez J, Mikulic M, Moreno P, Palacios I: Immediate and long-term outcome of percutaneous mitral balloon valvotomy in patients with mitral stenosis and atrial fibrillation. J Am Coll Cardiol 1999;34:1145–1152.
30 Davidson CJ, Bashore TM, Mickel M, et al: Balloon mitral commissurotomy after previous surgical commissurotomy. Circulation 1992;86:91–99.
31 Jang IK, Block PC, Newell JB, Tuzcu EM, Palacios IF: Percutaneous mitral balloon valvotomy for recurrent mitral stenosis after surgical commissurotomy. Am J Cardiol 1995;75:601–605.
32 Chen MH, Semigran M, Schwammenthal E, Harrell L, Palacios IF: Impact of pulmonary resistance on short- and long-term outcome after percutaneous mitral valvuloplasty. Circulation 1993(suppl I):1825.
33 Sagie A, Schwammenthal E, Newell JB, Harrell L, Weyman AE, Levine RA, Palacios IF: Significant tricuspid regurgitation is a marker for adverse outcome in patients undergoing mitral balloon valvotomy. J Am Coll Cardiol 1994;24:696–702.
34 Lopez-Cuellar JC, Leon MN, Pathan A, Mahdi NA, Simosa H, McMellon C, Harrell LC, Palacios IF: Ten-year follow-up of optimal candidates for percutaneous mitral balloon valvuloplasty. Circulation 1997;96(suppl I):2225.
35 Patel JJ, Sharma D, Mitha AS, Blyth D, Hassen F, Leroux BT, Sivabakiyam C: Balloon valvuloplasty versus closed commissurotomy for pliable mitral stenosis: A prospective hemodynamic study. J Am Coll Cardiol 1991;18:1318–1322.
36 Shrivastava S, Mathur A, Dev V, Saxena A, Venugopal P, Sampathkumar A: Comparison of immediate hemodynamic response of closed mitral commissurotomy, single-balloon and double-balloon mitral valvuloplasty in rheumatic mitral stenosis. J Thorac Cardiovasc Surg 1992;104:1264–1267.
37 Arora R, Nair M, Kalra GS, Nigam M, Khalilullah M. Immediate and long-term results of balloon and surgical closed mitral valvotomy: A randomized comparative study. Am Heart J 1993;125: 1091–1094.
38 Iung B, Cormier B, Ducimetiere P, Porte JM, Nallet O, Michel PL, Acar J, Vahanian A: Immediate results of percutaneous mitral commissurotomy. A predictive model on a series of 1514 patients. Circulation 1996;94:2124–2300.
39 Stefanadis CI, Stratos CG, Lambrou SG, Bahl VK, Cokkinos DV, Voudris VA, Foussas SG, Tsioufis CP, Toutouzas PK: Retrograde nontransseptal balloon mitral valvuloplasty: immediate results and intermediate long-term outcome in 441 cases – a multicenter experience. J Am Coll Cardiol 1998;32:1009–1016.
40 Chen CR, Cheng TO: Percutaneous balloon mitral valvuloplasty by the Inoue technique: a multicenter study of 4832 patients in China. Am Heart J 1995;129:1197–1203.
41 Multicenter experience with balloon mitral commissurotomy. NHLBI Balloon Valvuloplasty Registry Report on immediate and 30-day follow-up results. The National Heart, Lung, and Blood Institute Balloon Valvuloplasty Registry Participants. Circulation 1992;85:448–461.
42 Complications and mortality of percutaneous balloon mitral commissurotomy. A report from the National Heart, Lung, and Blood Institute Balloon Valvuloplasty Registry. Circulation 1992; 85: 2014–2024.
43 Ben Farhat M, Betbout F, Gamra H, Maatouk F, Ayari M, Cherif A, Jarrar M, Boussadia H, Hammami S, Chahbani I: Results of percutaneous double-balloon mitral commissurotomy in one medical center in Tunisia. Am J Cardiol 1995;76:1266–1270.
44 Arora R, Kalra GS, Murty GS, Trehan V, Jolly N, Mohan JC, Sethi KK, Nigam M, Khalilullah M: Percutaneous transatrial mitral commissurotomy: immediate and intermediate results. J Am Coll Cardiol 1994;23:1327–1332.
45 Cribier A, Eltchaninoff H, Koning R, Rath PC, Arora R, Imam A, El-Sayed M, Dani S, Derumeaux G, Benichou J, Tron C, Janorkar S, Pontier G, Letac B: Percutaneous mechanical mitral commissurotomy with a newly designed metallic valvulotome: immediate results of the initial experience in 153 patients. Circulation 1999;99:793–799.

Igor F. Palacios, MD, Cardiac Catheterization Laboratory and Interventional Cardiology,
Massachusetts General Hospital, Boston, MA 02114 (USA)
Tel. +1 617 7268424, E-Mail palacios.igor@mgh.harvard.edu

Borer JS, Isom OW (eds): Pathophysiology, Evaluation and Management of Valvular Heart Diseases.
Adv Cardiol. Basel, Karger, 2002, vol 39, pp 114–121

Mitral Commissurotomy and Valve Replacement for Mitral Stenosis: Observations on Selection of Surgical Procedures

O. Wayne Isom

Department of Cardiothoracic Surgery, and The Howard Gilman Institute for Valvular Heart Diseases, Weill Medical College of Cornell University, New York-Presbyterian Hospital-New York Weill Cornell Medical Center, New York, N.Y., USA

Mitral Commissurotomy: Closed and Open

Several approaches now exist for mechanical therapy for patients with mitral stenosis (MS). My personal opinion is heavily colored by the fact that, despite the outstanding statistics presented by Dr. Palacios elsewhere in this volume relating to catheter-based balloon valvular dilatation, as a surgeon I commonly see patients when the balloon procedure fails. I reoperate on several of these patients each year. Often, those that I see have required surgical intervention after 2–3 years of apparent success. Of course, I would not expect to see patients whose procedures are fully successful, but I have seen a sufficient number of failures to have formed some opinions about the mechanisms by which balloon dilatations achieve their successes, why they may fail, and why one might choose direct surgical valve repair or replacement as primary therapy in specific situations.

Though I favor primary surgical intervention for MS in many situations, I believe that, in this country today, there is no basis for performance of closed mitral commissurotomy (CMC) [1]. CMC was developed in another era, before availability of cardiopulmonary bypass, and was an important tool at a time when cardiopulmonary bypass was relatively primitive. This is no longer the case: the pump is safe. In addition, there are very few surgeons still in practice who are familiar with the necessary techniques and virtually none who apply them. The experts of earlier eras now are dead. Therefore, if CMC were to be performed, success would be far lower than when the procedure was common. Moreover, at its best, CMC is a very, very crude operation. It involves a lateral thoracotomy and a purse-string suture applied around the left atrial appendage. In addition, we previously demonstrated that left atrial thrombi are present in approximately 25% of surgical candidates for this procedure [2] and, since the CMC is performed without direct visualization of the interior of the left atrium, there is an important risk of stroke associated with accidental embolization during the operation. Given this background, the incidence of stroke Dr. Palacios's series seems particularly low at 1–2%.

From the experience with CMC, we and others long ago concluded that open mitral commissurotomy (OMC) is the preferable surgical approach. When this technique is applied, the peri-operative mortality is lower than that reported for balloon valvulotomy. Thus, we reported 0% mortality in 100 consecutive OMC in the *Journal of Thoracic Cardiovascular Surgery* over 25 years ago [2]. You should never lose a patient with MS who undergoes an OMC. In fact, when you open the atrium and actually look at the anatomy of the stenotic mitral valve, it is amazing that the CMC achieves any success at all. When rheumatic MS is present, the mitral commissures have grown together; the only way you relieve the stenosis is to split the valve; you do not split the commissures. In a patient on whom I recently operated after an unsuccessful balloon valvuloplasty, the balloon had ruptured the posterior mitral leaflet, in effect creating a three-cusp valve. This alleviated some of the MS, but the patient had insidiously developed mitral insufficiency (MR) during the ensuing 3 years. The fusion of the commissures involves dense fibrosis; splitting the commissures to achieve more physiological valve opening is virtually impossible. Therefore, it is not surprising that I have not seen any of the balloon dilatations split the mitral commissure. However, the dilatation device regularly succeeds in stretching the annulus, though the commissure remains fused. Therefore, I believe that, while balloon dilatation may be most appropriate for a patient at high peri-operative risk for some other reason (e.g., renal insufficiency) or for whom cardiopulmonary bypass involves particular hazard (e.g., because of a calcified aorta), at present, at least in the USA, I don't think there is a place for CMC, and only a limited role for balloon dilatation when standard surgical procedures and experienced surgical teams are available.

Mitral Valve Replacement: Artificial versus Biological Prostheses

While selection of surgical procedures is based partially and importantly on objective data, inter-patient variability is sufficiently great so that experience and clinical judgment are equally important. Therefore, I will present my opinions about procedure selection for patients with MS based on more than 25 years of surgical experience. Important considerations are presented below.

Age. As mentioned in Dr. Gardner's article elsewhere in this volume, age is a primary selection factor in choosing an artificial prosthesis versus a bioprosthesis. Dr. Gardner suggested that, from current data, age 65 may be a reasonable cut point for selection, with patients older than 65 years receiving bioprostheses. I look at patients in terms both of chronological age and physiological age. About 15–20 years ago, given the usual post-operative natural course, I would suggest that if a patient was >65 years old, expected life-span was markedly limited, and the tissue valve probably would outlive the patient, justifying its use. Now, I have had considerable experience with patients who received bioprostheses at age 70 and who have returned at 85 and 90 years of age with prosthetic failures, requiring reoperation. Conversely, we have all seen patients who are old at age 40. More commonly, though, we are now seeing patients in their 80s and above who may have normal or only modestly abnormal coronary arteries and capacity for wide-ranging activity. For these patients, tissue valves may be optimal. I have several patients who have received such valves in their 90s who were able to return to work without the lifestyle-limiting effects of anticoagulation. Therefore, I evaluate patients physiologically rather than chronologically.

Expected Lifestyle. Desired and expected future activity must be considered in selecting a valve, irrespective of expected valve survival. I operated on a policeman here in New York who wanted a porcine valve so that he could continue in his profession, which would have been precluded by anticoagulation. I have put three bioprostheses in this man over the past 30 years; each has lasted about 10 or 12 years. Similarly, if a patient expects to play contact sports, the need for anticoagulation precludes implantation of currently available artificial prostheses.

Cardiac Rhythm. If a patient is in chronic atrial fibrillation (AF) and unlikely to be convertible, lifelong anticoagulation is required; in this setting, there is no benefit to a tissue prosthesis but important benefit, in terms of valve survival, in using an artificial prosthesis. As a caveat, however, it must be noted that the chronicity of AF may be importantly altered by new surgical techniques, the application of which also may later influence valve selection. Increasing experience is being reported with operative ablation of AF pathways, the Maze procedure, and guidelines for application of this procedure now are being developed. If the left atrium >7 cm, ablation is unlikely to result in permanent restitution of sinus rhythm irrespective of early post-operative rhythm status. No benefit accrues to using a tissue valve in such a patient.

Status of Other Valves. The status of the other valves is another important factor in selection of the correct prosthesis for the mitral position. When the etiological process is rheumatic, though isolated rheumatic aortic valve disease can occur, it is highly uncommon. Almost always, the mitral valve also is involved.

Therefore, if operation is required in a younger person and you are going to replace the aortic valve with a mechanical prosthesis, you gain little by considering repair of the concomitantly diseased mitral valve, or use of a tissue prosthesis, since anticoagulants will be necessary.

Ventricular Function. One hears frequently about the importance of preservation of the subvalvular apparatus and the chordal attachments. In a patient with severely depressed ventricular function, these factors may have an influence on longevity and, thus, a tissue valve may present advantages.

Concomitant Coronary Disease. In the patients presenting in recent years, I do not see very much single vessel or double vessel disease. These patients usually are complex, having had several angioplasties with or without stents. Stents can present a major impediment to optimal surgical technique. I would appeal to cardiologists to send the patient to the surgeon before placing a stent far distally in the left anterior descending coronary artery. Distal stents leave no more than a centimeter in which to place the distal anastomosis of a bypass graft, an almost impossible situation for bypass grafting, known as 'the full metal jacket' to our residents. If a patient has severe coronary disease requiring 4 or 5 grafts as well as operable mitral valve disease, it may be best to replace the valve and reduce cardiopulmonary bypass time, rather than considering a repair procedure.

Status of the Other Bodily Systems. If there is a history of peptic ulcer disease or any type of gastrointestinal bleeding, it is preferable to avoid anticoagulation. Hematological problems, particularly coagulopathies, should lead to avoidance of artificial valves. Patients on chronic renal dialysis seem to manifest prominent calcification of tissue valves. Neurological and pulmonary conditions can influence appropriateness of anticoagulation, as well.

Patient Compliance. I think New Yorkers are pretty sophisticated. They go to the doctor fairly often. However, if the patient lives in the woods of East Texas, he is not going to come back to see the doctor for a year, perhaps by culture or choice but more likely because of logistic inconvenience. The latter patient is not a candidate for anticoagulation or for an artificial prosthesis. For the surgeon, determination of compliance requires close communication with the internist or cardiologist who is most familiar with the patient's personality and history.

Peri-Operative Mortality, Prosthesis Durability and Long-Term Morbidity. With OMC, in appropriately selected patients, that is, those who are <35 years old, with little calcification, 25 event-free years should be expected. Even with CMC, when done properly, and even though CMC is a blind procedure, 25 event-free years was not unusual. The mortality for an OMC in a patient without coronary disease ought to be 0% and the incidence of stroke ought to be $<1\%$, especially in those <35 years old. At a reputable center with a reputable surgeon, that is what should be expected.

Observations on Surgical Techniques

In terms of surgical technique, whenever possible you should preserve the mitral valve, with annuloplasty when necessary. The advances in annuloplasty with a ring has been a great benefit in enhancing long-term results. I learned how to do a mitral annuloplasty from George Reed who had done several in the 1960s on rheumatic patients. He called the procedure an exaggerated asymmetric annuloplasty [3]. It worked beautifully because the tissue was very good. When we began operating on 'floppy' valves, especially those with a ruptured chordae, excellent results were obtained in only about 75%; 25% recurred, attributable to a dilated annulus. After Duran et al. [4] introduced the use of a prosthetic ring in the mid-1970s to decrease the size of the annulus, results improved dramatically. Therefore, when possible, preservation of the valve and its normal architecture is highly desirable. However, I must offer an important caveat: though I can repair any valve, if I repair a valve and the patient returns in a year or two with another ruptured chord, the patient will be justifiably dissatisfied with me – and with the cardiologist who provided the referral! For example, if a patient is in AF and the chordae all are long and attenuated, then long-term stability with repair may be suboptimal and the advantage of preclusion of anticoagulation is likely to be lost; in this situation, replacement may be preferable. Unfortunately, prior to surgery echocardiography cannot fully define the appearance and character of the chordae. At operation, if I find they are particularly thin and attenuated, though I can shorten them, I need to employ some judgment regarding the likelihood that a stable long-term repair can be achieved; replacement may be the better decision in this setting. As with OMC, the peri-operative mortality and major morbidity associated with annuloplasty should be 0 and <1%, respectively, and one should be aiming for at least 20–25 years of stable valve function.

The various tissue valve options are reviewed elsewhere in this volume by Dr. Gardner. I will not repeat the full range of choices. However, it is worth noting that, generically, tissue valves can be either relatively intact porcine valves or prostheses constructed from bovine pericardium. The story of the development of these valves is interesting. The problem with tissue valve homografts was to determine an appropriate source. For this, in essence, you need to make a deal with the local undertaker. Barrett-Boyes in New Zealand had such an arrangement; he had the local undertakers call him as soon as they were called about a death. For this, he gave them a fifth of scotch every Christmas, and received fresh valves. You cannot do that in this country. However, this problem interested Hancock, a chemist at the NIH. He decided that the pig valve was about the same size as the human valve and that all that was necessary to make it serviceable was a way to preserve it while maintaining the structural integrity of the valve, and destroying the antigenicity and sterilizing it at the same time. In the late 1960s he conceived of using formaldehyde, the same preservative used for specimens in colleges and medical schools. He preserved a large number of pig valves with a dilute solution of formaldehyde. Several of these were inserted in operations at Mount Sinai Hospital in New York in the late 1960s, but the result was catastrophic. The heterografts calcified within 6–18 months and needed to be removed. Hancock developed the idea of fixation with glutaraldehyde, which differs from formaldehyde by 1 carbon atom but has many of the same properties. This worked. It produced less ultrastructural change than formaldehyde: by electron microscopy, collagen cross-linkages were preserved to a greater extent. That was the beginning of valve heterografting. At the time, nobody knew whether it was going to work, but it did! Sometime thereafter, in an archeological study, it was reported that 0.25% glutaraldehyde was found in Egyptian mummies that were very well preserved, so maybe nothing is new under the sun!

There are two types of porcine valves, Hancock and Edwards. Most experience has been with the mounted porcine prosthesis, involving a pig aortic valve mounted within an artificial sewing ring to facilitate suturing the valve in place. However, early experience with unmounted valves, attached free-hand, suggests that this approach results in greater valve flexibility. Unmounted valves continue to be used, and several surgeons believe they provide enhanced long-term results compared with the mounted prostheses. I think it is too early to tell whether the free-hand approach truly improves results. All porcine valves can be expected to last 10–15 years, though some fail earlier and some remain viable for considerably longer. Of those I have personally inserted, the longest duration of viability has been 24 years; several now are at 17 or 18 years and still functioning well. However, I usually tell a patient that if we use a porcine valve, it will last between 10 and 15 years, the usual range with a tissue valve in the mitral position.

Early experiences with the bovine pericardial valve in Europe indicated good 14-year durability. However, at present, I think it is appropriate to indicate to the patient that, while more than 15 years of use may be possible, 10–15 years is the most realistic expectation, after which tissue valves, particularly in the mitral position, do wear out.

For isolated mitral valve replacement, if function of the left and right ventricles is well preserved and there is no associated coronary disease, peri-operative mortality should be <1%; even with associated problems, if the mitral valve disease is non-ischemic, <2% peri-operative mortality should be expected [5]. These values are achieved in our program. If coronary disease and ventricular dysfunction are present (we are now operating on patients with left ventricular ejection fractions as low as 15–20%), survival can be improved compared with medical treatment alone, but peri-operative mortality clearly is increased. Long-term, the morbidity associated with the tissue valve should be essentially the incidence of bacterial endocarditis, since anticoagulation is not required. It is important to remember that patients with tissue valves require infective endocarditis prophylaxis since the valve is a foreign body.

When tissue valves fail, in most instances dysfunction occurs insidiously over a long period, not suddenly. Occasionally, acute rupture of one of the struts occurs and represents an emergency, but this is highly uncommon. In routine use, annual echocardiograms to seek MR and calcification provide considerable time for decisions about appropriateness of re-replacement.

Among the artificial prostheses, the ball valve, first used in the 1950s and perfected by Starr in the mid-1960s, now is largely of historical interest though many were used [6]. Starr is still in active practice. He told me about his original experimental studies with the ball valve with replacement in cows or calves. One of the key problems was the thrombogenicity of the prosthesis: despite anticoagulation, the valves all clotted off in the calves. Starr then determined that calves intrinsically were more thrombogenic than humans and began inserting them in humans ... and they worked. However, I do not think we could follow this development pathway for a new valve today. The tilting disc valve was an improvement hemodynamically but problems developed with this prosthesis as well. However, with additional development, the pivoting disc valve was produced. This valve type has been used since the mid-1970s, with several million exposures. There are three different types and, essentially, they are probably all about the same. Initially, I believed that one was more thrombogenic in the mitral position than another, but in a recent study presented at the American Association of Thoracic Surgery this year [7], no difference in thrombotic complications was reported among the valve types in a large group of patients with reasonable follow-up.

From the surgeon's perspective, sewing rings differ modestly. This can be an important consideration in prosthesis selection, particularly when patient presentation is unusual. In a patient who has a myocardial infarction and a rupture of the papillary muscle, in whom the posterior wall of the heart is very, very friable with the consistency of warm butter, a slight enhancement in sewing ring pliability can be an extraordinary advantage in achieving a stable valve implantation.

Conclusions

In summary, in selecting approaches to surgical/mechanical therapy for patients with MS (or with any mitral pathology), large group follow-up data are very important, but intra-patient variation is large. Therefore, look at the patient as a whole, talk to the cardiologist, talk to the internist, talk to the family, and try to match that patient with the therapy.

References

1 Isom OW, Shemin RJ, Whiddon LL: Rheumatic mitral valve disease; in Glenn W (ed): Thoracic and Cardiovascular Surgery, ed 4. New York, Prentice-Hall, 1982.

2 Mullin MJ, Engelman RM, Isom OW, Boyd AD, Glassman E, Spencer FC: Experience with open mitral commissurotomy in 100 consecutive patients. Surgery 1974;76:974–982.

3 Reed GE, Tice DA, Clauss RH: Asymmetric exaggerated mitral annuloplasty: Repair of mitral insufficiency with hemodynamic predictability. J Thorac Cardiovasc Surg 1965;49:752–760.

4 Duran CG, Pomar JL, Revuelta JM, Gallo I, Poveda J, Ochoteco A, Ubago JL: Conservative operation for mitral insufficiency. J Thorac Cardiovasc Surg 1980;79:326–332.

5 Borer JS, Supino P, Hochreiter C, Herrold EM, Yin A, Swan C, Krieger K, Isom OW: Effect of coronary artery bypass grafting on fatal and non-fatal complications early after surgery for non-ischemic valvular heart disease and associated coronary artery disease; in Lewis BS, Halon DA, Flugelman MY, Hradec J (eds): Advances in Coronary Artery Disease. Proc 4th Int Congr Coronary Artery Disease. Bologna, Monduzzi, 2001, pp 119–125.

6 Isom OW, Spencer FC, Glassman E, Teiko P, Boyd AD, Cunningham JN, Reed GE: Long-term results in 1,375 patients undergoing valve replacement with Starr-Edwards cloth-covered steel ball prostheses. Ann Surg 1977;186:310–323.

7 Lim KHH, Caputo M, Ascione R, Wild JM, West R, Angielini GD, Bryan AJ: A prospective randomized comparison of CarboMedics and St Judes medical mechanical heart valve prosthesis: An interim report. Proc 81st Annual Meeting of the American Association for Thoracic Surgery, 2001, p 54.

O. Wayne Isom, MD, Department of Cardiothoracic Surgery, New York Weill Cornell Medical Center, 525 East 68th Street, New York, NY 10021 (USA)

Borer JS, Isom OW (eds): Pathophysiology, Evaluation and Management of Valvular Heart Diseases.
Adv Cardiol. Basel, Karger, 2002, vol 39, pp 122–129

Mitral Regurgitation: Natural History in Operated and Unoperated Patients

Clare A. Hochreiter, Jeffrey S. Borer, Edmund McM. Herrold, Phyllis G. Supino, Karl H. Krieger, O. Wayne Isom

Division of Cardiovascular Pathophysiology, Department of Cardiothoracic Surgery and The Howard Gilman Institute for Valvular Heart Diseases, Weill Medical College of Cornell University, New York, N.Y., USA

Accurate and complete knowledge of the natural history of patients with non-ischemic mitral regurgitation (MR) would be a tremendous aid in the management of patients with this disease. Unfortunately, our knowledge in this area is limited because in the era before surgical intervention was available and was applied to alter natural history, long-term epidemiological studies using sequential objective imaging techniques were not performed. As a result, the natural history of cardiac performed is not known for the full course of the disease. In addition, until recently, little information has been available defining clinical or objective disease progression in asymptomatic patients. However, in recent years we and others have evaluated the natural history of cardiac function and clinical debility in patients with MR to enhance our knowledge of the spectrum of this disease. This paper will outline our current understanding of the natural history of the patient with MR.

Surgical intervention for MR was introduced about 40 years ago. At that time, detailed non-invasive evaluation of patients with suspected MR was not yet available. Due to an initial high mortality risk, surgery was first applied only in severely symptomatic patients. However, as surgical techniques have advanced, surgical correction of MR has become an option for less symptomatic and even asymptomatic patients. At no time has there been a randomized study to compare the natural history of either symptomatic or asymptomatic patients with well-characterized MR who were assigned to either medical or surgical therapy.

The natural history of patients with MR can be analyzed for two distinct groups: (1) patients who have not had surgical intervention and (2) patients who have undergone surgical correction of MR. For each group, both patient survival and the natural history of ventricular function have been reported.

Unoperated Patients: Survival

In 1975, Rapaport [1] reported an 80% 5-year survival and a 60% 10-year survival in medically treated patients with MR. Although not specifically stated, we can probably assume that these patients varied from asymptomatic to moderately symptomatic on medical therapy since surgery was available only for patients with severe symptoms. There was no invasive or non-invasive assessment of ventricular function or of MR severity reported for these patients. At about the same time, Hammermeister et al. [2] reported a much more ominous survival in his unoperated medically treated cohort: 5-year survival was 55% and 10-year survival was only 20% for patients with isolated MR. In this later retrospective study, all patients had undergone cardiac catheterization and thus, the majority of patients were probably FC III or IV with severe MR. However, neither functional class nor ventricular function measurements were reported specifically for the subset of patients with isolated MR.

Subsequent studies help to reconcile these discrepant findings. In 1984, Ramanathan et al. [3] also reported survival in medically treated patients. Here, the overall 5-year survival was approximately 70%, intermediate between the Rapaport and Hammermeister results. Additional data in Ramanathan's report allows estimation for a 4-year survival of over 80% in those patients with absent or relatively mild symptoms (class I–II), similar to the survival in Rapaport's more optimistic report, whereas those with severe symptoms had an approximately 55% 4-year survival, similar to the report of Hammermeister. Thus, symptom status was identified early as an important predictor of natural history in patients with unoperated MR.

In a prospective study by our group [4], reported in 1986, it became clear that survival in medically treated patients was also strongly linked to ventricular function, with the short-term survival being extremely poor in those patients with subnormal left (LV) and/or right ventricular (RV) function regardless of symptoms (fig. 1). However, the majority of deaths were sudden, rather than from progressive heart failure. Thus, prognosis is poor for patients with unoperated severe MR if they manifest either severe symptoms or reduced ventricular function. Importantly, RV function tended to be more predictive than LV function in our patients. RV function was inversely related to pulmonary artery pressure and treadmill exercise tolerance, providing a probable link between RV function

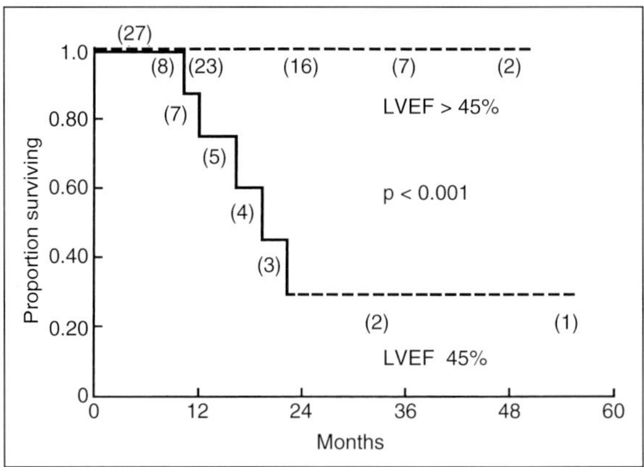

Fig. 1. MR: medically treated patients [from 4, with permission].

and symptoms (no such relation was apparent between exercise tolerance and LV function [4]). However, the prognosis for unoperated patients with symptoms but normal ventricular function has not been well defined.

The natural history of predominantly asymptomatic patients with moderate to severe MR due to mitral valve prolapse, with normal RV and LV function, was reported from a prospective study by Rosen [5], of our group, in 1994. Prognosis was much more benign in this group than among symptomatic patients. During nearly 5 years (average) of follow-up, there were no deaths and no progression to subnormal ventricular function, but there was a 10% average annual risk of developing symptoms leading to surgery. Importantly, these patients could be dichotomized with regard to the effect of exercise on RV function into relatively low risk (4% per year) and relatively high risk (14% per year) for progression to symptoms of heart failure.

Unoperated Patients: Natural History of Ventricular Function

To determine the natural history of ventricular function in unoperated patients with 3–4 + MR, we analyzed data on all patients in our prospectively studied population who had at least three serial echocardiograms and/or radionuclide ventriculograms over at least 4 years [6]. In our preliminary report of these data, from a population including 35 asymptomatic or minimally symptomatic patients, each of whom underwent an average of six radionuclide studies and six echo studies, we found that the average rate of change was slow in ventricular size, atrial size, LV ejection fraction (EF) or RVEF. For example, our preliminary analysis [6] suggests that over a maximum follow-up of 12 years,

LVEF at rest falls <0.1% (EF units) per year, and LVEF during exercise falls <1% per year, while RVEF fall approaches 0.5% per year at rest and 1% per year during exercise. Among individual patients, the change was modest even in those with the most rapid progression. Of note, in any individual patient the variability in a single measurement from year to year often far exceeded the general trend in that measurement over several years, thus emphasizing the need to confirm any large change in either ventricular size or function before recommending a major treatment change such as surgery.

Operated Patients: Survival

There have been many reports of prognosis after surgical correction for MR. Most have relatively similar findings. Although most patients who survive surgical correction of MR have symptomatic improvement, some do not improve symptomatically and/or manifest poor late post-operative survival.

A major determinant of post-operative survival is pre-operative ventricular function. In 1981, Phillips et al. [7] reported a 90% 5-year post-operative survival for patients whose pre-operative LVEF was >50%, but only a 40% 5-year survival in those with a pre-operative LVEF <40%. In 1994, Enriquez-Sarano et al. [8] reported similar findings, with 10-year survival of 72% when pre-operative LVEF was ⩾60%. However, survival dropped to 32% if pre-operative LVEF was <50%.

Nevertheless, patients with subnormal EF still can benefit from surgery. Symptoms often improve, and survival also appears to improve. In a prospective but not randomized study, Wencker [9] of our group found that patients with subnormal RVEF and/or LVEF before operation had a better prognosis with surgical therapy than with medical therapy. In smaller subgroups matched for LVEF, survival in the surgical group remained better than in the unoperated medically treated group.

Pre-operative symptom status also has an important impact on post-operative survival. Tribouilloy et al. [10] reported 76% 10-year post-operative survival in patients in NYHA FC I–II before operation compared with 48% in those who were in FC III–IV pre-operatively. This finding has been seen consistently in multiple reports. Pre-operative symptom status is a predictor of post-operative prognosis regardless of the pre-operative EF or the type surgical correction (repair or replacement) performed.

Somewhat less certain is the effect of mitral valve repair compared to mitral valve replacement on the natural history of patients who undergo surgical correction of MR. Those patients who are eligible or selected for mitral valve repair often differ in terms of symptoms, ventricular function and age compared

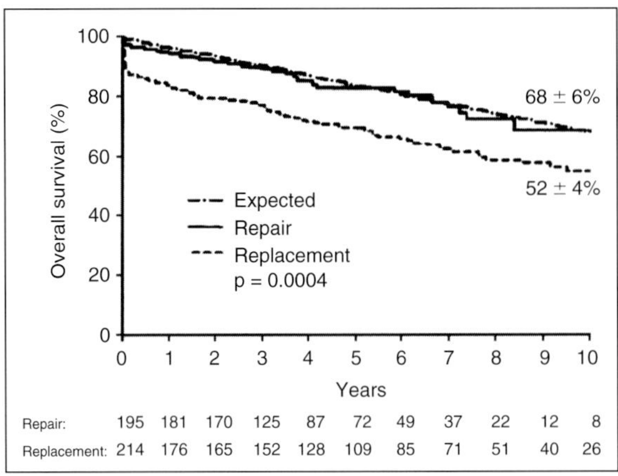

Fig. 2. MR: post-operative outcome [from 13, with permission].

with those who undergo replacement. Despite trying to control for this bias, which would generally favor improved survival in patients undergoing repair, studies have reached differing conclusions. Studies by Galloway et al. [11] and Carver et al. [12] failed to show any difference in survival with respect to repair versus replacement in a multivariate analysis or when patients were matched for important pre-operative variables. However, a recent large study from Enriquez-Sarano et al. [13], using a multivariate model, found that survival after repair was improved compared with replacement. In the repair group, survival was similar to that expected in the general population, while survival in the replacement group was not as favorable (fig. 2). However, one of the major differences affecting late post-operative survival was the higher operative mortality in the replacement group in this study.

Operative mortality remains a factor in overall late mortality after surgical repair of MR. Operative/peri-operative mortality for surgical correction of MR has decreased over time due to improved surgical care and the trend toward operating on younger patients when disease is less advanced and more likely to be amendable to repair rather than replacement. Most large centers have reduced the overall operative mortality for pure, isolated MR to <3%. Besides age, which is likely a marker for comorbid disease, other factors which influence operative mortality are functional class, year of surgery, prior cardiac surgery and need for concomitant coronary bypass surgery.

Many studies have found that late after surgical correction of MR, death often is sudden. Thus, the natural history of operated patients also may be importantly affected by ventricular arrhythmias. In our prospective study [14], 24-hour ambulatory ECGs were done routinely in all MR patients at yearly intervals.

In a preliminary report [14] of 53 operated patients who had 24-hour ambulatory ECGs both before and after surgery, there were 8 late post-operative cardiac deaths, 5 of which were sudden. Sudden death after surgery was found only in those patients who had non-sustained ventricular tachycardia (defined as ⩾3 consecutive VPCs) on at least one of their post-operative ambulatory ECGs. Not surprisingly, the risk of sudden death was highest in those patients with non-sustained ventricular tachycardia and subnormal ventricular function. However, several sudden deaths occurred in patients who were asymptomatic with normal ventricular function after their MV surgery. Further study in this area is needed to determine if any additional diagnostic tests can identify which patients with asymptomatic ventricular arrhythmias are at highest risk and whether any specific anti-arrhythmia therapies can improve late post-operative prognosis.

Operated Patients: Natural History of Ventricular Function

Though many studies have evaluated the effect of valve replacement or repair on early post-operative ventricular function, the natural history of ventricular function late after mitral valve surgery has not been extensively studied. Most early post-operative studies have found a fall in LVEF of about 10% early after mitral valve replacement. This fall generally is less marked, or even absent, in patients who have undergone repair. Only a few small studies have reported ventricular function late after surgery. In studies by both Boucher et al. [15] and Starling et al. [16], there was modest improvement in LVEF in many but not all patients late after surgery compared with the initial postoperative decrease in LVEF. Although there was some overlap, late improvement in LVEF was more common in patients with normal preoperative LVEF.

Preliminary results from our prospectively followed patients reveal late improvement in exercise LVEF after either repair or replacement. However, on average, late improvement in resting function was small. RVEF, depressed before operation (largely by pressure loading rather than volume loading) usually rebounds markedly early after operation and maintains this improvement in subsequent years [17].

Conclusions

The natural history of patients with MR is not completely understood. However, recent studies suggest relatively slow objective progression and moderately slow symptom progression in asymptomatic patients, while post-operative outcome is strongly related to pre-operative symptom and RV and LV function status. Our conclusions are summarized in table 1.

Table 1. Natural history of patients with MR

Unoperated patients
1. Survival is good in patients who are asymptomatic with normal ventricular function
2. Progressive changes in LV size and function generally are slow
3. Symptoms most often develop before nominal ventricular dysfunction; however, both require frequent monitoring
4. Survival falls when either RV or LV function becomes subnormal

Operated patients
1. Survival after surgical correction of MR is strongly related to pre-operative ventricular function and symptoms
2. MV repair may offer several advantages compared to MV replacement but its role in improving survival remains uncertain, and probably depends in part on the characteristics of the operated cohort
3. LV function generally decreases early after MV surgery but at later follow-up some modest functional recovery may be seen; RV function generally improves quickly following MV surgery
4. Sudden death late after MV surgery is associated with non-sustained ventricular tachycardia and ventricular dysfunction. Further studies are needed to identify those at high risk and to devise treatments to improve post-operative survival

Acknowledgements

Dr. Borer is the Gladys and Roland Harriman Professor of Cardiovascular Medicine at Cornell and was supported in part during this work by an endowment from the Gladys and Roland Harriman Foundation, New York, N.Y. In addition, the work reported herein was supported in part by National Heart Lung and Blood Institute, Bethesda, Md. (RO1- HL-26504), and by grants from The Howard Gilman Foundation, New York, N.Y., The Schiavone Family Foundation, White House Station, N.J., The Charles and Jean Brunie Foundation, Bronxville, N.Y., The David Margolis Foundation, New York, N.Y., The American Cardio-Vascular Research Foundation, New York, N.Y., The Irving R. Hansen Foundation, New York, N.Y., The Mary A.H. Rumsey Foundation, New York, N.Y., The Messinger Family Foundation, New York, N.Y., The Daniel and Elaine Sargent Charitable Trust, New York, N.Y., The A.C. Israel Foundation, Greenwich, Conn., and by much appreciated gifts from Maryjane and the late William Voute, Bronxville, N.Y., and Stephen and Suzanne Weiss, Greenwich, Conn.

References

1 Rapaport E: Natural history of aortic and mitral valve disease. Am J Cardiol 1975;35:221–227.

2 Hammermeister KE, Fisher L, Kennedy W, Samuels S, Dodge H: Prediction of late survival in patients with mitral disease from clinical, hemodynamic and quantitative angiographic variables. Circulation 1978;57:341–349.

3 Ramanathan KB, Knowles J, Conner MJ, Tribble R, Kroetz FW, Sullivan JM, Mirvis DM: Natural history of chronic mitral regurgitation: Relation of the peak systolic pressure/end systolic volume ratio to morbidity and mortality. J Am Coll Cardiol 1984;3:1412–1416.

4 Hochreiter C, Niles N, Devereux RB, Kligfield P, Borer JS: Mitral regurgitation: Relationship of noninvasive descriptors of right and left ventricular performance to clinical and hemodynamic findings and to prognosis in medically and surgically treated patients. Circulation 1986;73: 900–912.

5 Rosen SE, Borer JS, Hochreiter C, Supino P, Roman MJ, Devereux RB, Kligfield P, Bucek J: Natural history of asymptomatic/minimally symptomatic patients with severe mitral regurgitation secondary to mitral valve prolapse and normal right and left ventricular performance. Am J Cardiol 1994;74:374–380.

6 Hochreiter CA, Borer JS, Engel DA, Devereux RB, Roman MJ, Kligfield PD, Herrold EM, Supino PG, Bergstein NI. Natural history of right and left ventricular size and function in patients with asymptomatic chronic severe non-ischemic mitral regurgitation. J Am Coll Cardiol 2000;35:2: 1001–171:524A.

7 Phillips HR, Levine FH, Carter JE, Boucher CA, Osbakken MD, Okada RD, Akins CW, Daggett WM, Buckley MJ, Pohost GM: Mitral valve replacement for isolate mitral regurgitation: Analysis of clinical course and late post-operative left ventricular ejection fraction. Am J Cardiol 1981;48:647–654.

8 Enriquez-Sarano M, Tajik AJ, Schaff HV, Orszulak TA, Bailey KR, Frye RL: Echocardiographic prediction of survival after surgical correction of organic mitral regurgitation. Circulation 1994; 90:830–837.

9 Wencker D, Borer JS, Hochreiter C, Devereux RB, Roman MJ, Kligfield P, Supino P, Krieger K, Isom OW: Preoperative predictors of late postoperative outcome among patients with nonischemic mitral regurgitation with 'high risk' descriptors and comparison with unoperated patients. Cardiology 2000;93:37–42.

10 Tribouilloy CM, Enriquez-Sarano M, Schaff HV, Orszulak TA, Bailey KR, Tajik AJ, Frye RL: Impact of preoperative symptoms on survival after surgical correction of organic mitral regurgitation. Rational for optimizing surgical indication. Circulation 1999;99:400–405.

11 Galloway AC, Colvin SB, Baumann FG, Grossi EA, Ribakove GH, Harty S, Spencer FC: A comparison of mitral valve reconstruction with mitral valve replacement: intermediate-term results. Ann Thorac Surg 1989;47:655–662.

12 Carver JM, Cohen C, Weintraub WS: Case-matched comparison of mitral valve replacement and repair. Ann Thorac Surg 1990;49:964–969.

13 Enriquez-Sarano M, Schaff HV, Orszulak TA, Tajik AJ, Bailey KR, Frye RL: Valve repair improves the outcome of surgery for mitral regurgitation. A multivariate analysis. Circulation 1995;91: 1022–1028.

14 Hochreiter CA, Borer JS, Supino PG, Herrold EM, Kligfield PD, Bergstein NI, Krieger K, Isom OW: Ventricular arrhythmias and sudden death after surgery for chronic non-ischemic mitral regurgitation. Circulation 2000;102(suppl II):369.

15 Boucher CA, Birgham JB, Osbakken MD, Okada RD, Strauss HW, Block PC, Levine FH, Phillips HR, Pohost GM: Early changes in left ventricular size and function after correction of left ventricular volume overload. Am J Cardiol 1981;47:991–1004.

16 Starling MR, Kirsh MM, Montgomery DG, Gross MD: Impaired left ventricular contractile function in patients with long-term mitral regurgitation and normal ejection fraction. J Am Coll Cardiol 1993;22:239–250.

17 Wencker D, Borer JS, Hochreiter C, Devereux RB, Roman MJ, Kligfield P, Supino P: Radionuclide-based selection for mitral surgery in high-risk patients with non-ischemic mitral regurgitation. J Nucl Cardiol 1997;4:S60.

Jeffrey S. Borer, MD, Division of Cardiovascular Pathophysiology,
New York-Presbyterian Hospital, New York Weill Cornell Center,
525 East 68th Street, New York, NY 10021 (USA)

Borer JS, Isom OW (eds): Pathophysiology, Evaluation and Management of Valvular Heart Diseases.
Adv Cardiol. Basel, Karger, 2002, vol 39, pp 130–132

Complications of Mitral Valve Prolapse

Robert M. Jeresaty

Division of Cardiology, St. Francis Hospital and Medical Center,
University of Connecticut School of Medicine, Hartford, Conn., USA

Mitral valve prolapse (MVP) is a common cardiac disorder [1–5]. A 5% prevalence has been reported in previous reviews. In November 1999, on the basis of strict echocardiographic criteria, the Framingham Heart Study reported a 2–4% prevalence in the general population. This finding of a lower prevalence of MVP than previously reported has been widely disseminated in the media. I submit that a valvular disorder that affects 2–4% of the population is still the most common cardiac valvular abnormality in industrialized countries. The Framingham Heart Study deserves credit for demonstrating that chest pain and dyspnea are not more common in subjects with MVP than in subjects without prolapse and that the previously reported association was probably due to a selection bias. The emphasis should switch from the so-called 'MVP syndrome' to the mitral valvular complications of MVP.

The prognosis of MVP is generally favorable. Its course may be infrequently complicated by progression of mitral regurgitation (MR), ruptured chordae tendineae, endocarditis, transient ischemic attacks and sudden death. Considering the high prevalence of MVP and the relative rare occurrence of complications, we must infer that MVP has a generally benign course. Patients with MVP associated with a murmur of MR, men, and individuals with thickened and redundant leaflets on echocardiography, are at greatest risk of developing complications. In all probability, patients who develop a regurgitant murmur have already demonstrated a progressive tendency. The complications of MVP are listed and discussed below.

MR: Development and Progression

It is generally accepted that MVP is the most common cause of severe pure MR in developed countries which have witnessed an almost complete extinction of acute rheumatic fever. In developing countries, rheumatic heart disease remains the major cause of MR. Most patients with MVP and severe MR are men in their 60s and 70s. We and others have followed patients with clicks and murmurs who have subsequently developed severe MR, with or without ruptured chordae. The aging of the population allows the development of MR, which becomes evident in the elderly. Moreover MVP is presently diagnosed accurately and is no longer confused with rheumatic heart disease. Mitral valve repair has had a major beneficial effect on the prognosis of MVP associated with MR. Among the causes of MR, MVP is the most amenable to repair and is associated with the highest freedom from operation.

Ruptured Chordae Tendineae

Ruptured chordae tendineae have been accepted as a major complication of MVP. We and others have demonstrated an etiological link between MVP and ruptured chordae. With the help of Dr. Jesse Edwards, the well-known pathologist, we examined the valves of 25 patients with ruptured chordae who underwent mitral valve replacement [4]. In our series, MVP was the underlying pathologic abnormality in 23 patients (92%), endocarditis in the absence of MVP in 1 patient, and valvular abnormality was unknown in 1 patient. Of the 23 patients with underlying MVP, 2 had endocarditis, but in only 1 of the 2, endocarditis could be held historically and pathologically responsible for the chordal rupture. We and others have documented the occurrence of chordal rupture in at least 40 patients previously diagnosed as classical MVP by auscultatory and echocardiographic criteria. These patients provide a strong argument in favor of a causal relationship between MVP and ruptured chordae tendineae. Chordal rupture in MVP may be due to degeneration of collagen within the central core of the chordae or to increased chordal tension resulting from the enlarged area of the cusps. In view of the demonstration of MVP as the most frequent cause of ruptured chordae tendineae, the term 'idiopathic' should no longer be used to designate most cases of ruptured chordae tendineae.

Infective Endocarditis

Infective endocarditis is emerging as another major complication of MVP now that rheumatic heart disease has become uncommon in developed countries. It has been reported in MVP associated with regurgitant murmur but rarely in the silent form and in isolated clicks. Male sex, age >45 and thickening of mitral leaflets on echocardiography identify patients at increased risk of endocarditis. In these patients who are at high risk, endocarditis prophylaxis is warranted.

Transient Ischemic Attacks

Transient ischemic attacks and major strokes have been reported as a complication of MVP, particularly in the young. This etiologic association remains unproved and, if present, uncommon.

Sudden Death

Sudden death is the most feared, but fortunately, the most uncommon complication of MVP. About 200 cases have been reported. Ventricular fibrillation is believed to be the mechanism of sudden death in this valve disorder. A family history of sudden death due to MVP and/or history of syncope of probable arrhythmic origin are felt to be predictors of sudden death, warranting active investigation, antiarrhythmic management and, in selected cases, the insertion of automatic defibrillators.

Conclusion

In conclusion, despite its generally benign outlook and in view of its high prevalence, MVP accounts for most cases of severe MR, including 90% of the cases of ruptured chordae. It is the most commonly recognized lesion among adults with native valve endocarditis.

References

1 Freed LA, Levy D, Levine RA, et al: Prevalence and clinical outcome of mitral valve prolapse. N Engl J Med 1999;341:1–7.

2 Jeresaty RM: Mitral valve prolapse: An update. JAMA 1985;254:793–795.

3 Waller BF, Morrow AG, Maron BJ, et al: Etiology of clinically isolated, severe, chronic, pure mitral regurgitation: Analysis of 97 patients over 30 years of age having mitral valve replacement. Am Heart J 1982;104:276–288.

4 Jeresaty RM, Edwards JE, Chawla SK: Mitral valve prolapse and ruptured chordae tendineae. Am J Cardiol 1985;55:138–142.

5 McKinsey DS, Ratts TE, Bisno AL: Underlying cardiac lesions in adults with infective endocarditis: The changing spectrum. Am J Med 1987;82:681–688.

Robert M. Jeresaty, MD, St. Francis Hospital and Medical Center, Section of Cardiology,
114 Woodland Street, Hartford, CT 06105-1299 (USA)

Borer JS, Isom OW (eds): Pathophysiology, Evaluation and Management of Valvular Heart Diseases.
Adv Cardiol. Basel, Karger, 2002, vol 39, pp 133–143

Mitral Regurgitation: Predictors of Outcome and Natural History

Maurice Enriquez-Sarano[a], *Vuysile Nkomo*[b], *Dania Mohty*[b], *Jean-Francois Avierinos*[b], *Hari Chaliki*[b]

Divisions of [a] Cardiovascular Diseases and [b] Internal Medicine, Mayo Clinic and Mayo Foundation, Rochester, Minn., USA

Mitral regurgitation (MR) is a common valvular heart disease [1] which was long thought to be well-tolerated for many years and for which surgery was performed only when deterioration was clinically evident. With the regression of rheumatic disease and the aging of the population, degenerative MR with mitral valve prolapse (MVP) has become the major cause of organic MR [2, 3]. New data on the natural history of the disease, new methods of quantitation of MR, new observations on the benefits of valve repair (coupled with improving surgical repair techniques), and increasingly extensive utilization of intra-operative echocardiography have led to profound changes in the indications for surgery with widespread evolution towards earlier surgery in organic MR.

Natural History of Severe Mitral Regurgitation

Clinical Outcome of Severe MR. Previous literature reported widely disparate estimates of long-term survival in patients with MR, between 97 and 27% at 5 years [4, 5]. Analysis of the natural history of MR due to flail leaflets is important because 85% of patients with flail leaflets present with severe MR [6]. We observed that, in comparison to the expected survival, an excess mortality was noted (6.3% yearly) (fig. 1). A high morbidity was also present: over 10 years, 30% of patients develop atrial fibrillation, >65% develop heart failure, and 90% have undergone surgery or died. Therefore, in patients with severe MR, operation is almost unavoidable over 10 years of follow-up. Patients with class III or IV symptoms, even transient, displayed a considerable mortality (34% yearly) if

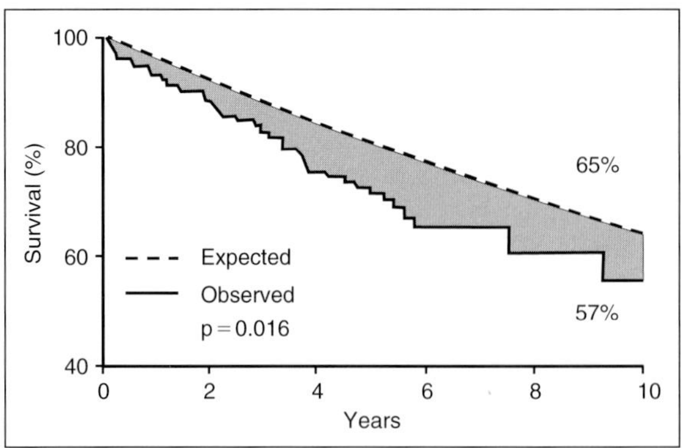

Fig. 1. Survival in patients with medically treated MR due to flail mitral leaflets. Note the excess mortality as compared to the expected survival (shaded area) [from 6, with permission].

not operated, but even those in class I or II had a notable mortality (4.1% yearly). Patients with left ventricular (LV) ejection fraction (EF) <60% also displayed an excess mortality as compared to those with LVEF ≥60%, but no group at very low risk under medical treatment could be defined.

Sudden death, a catastrophic event, accounts for approximately one quarter of deaths during medical treatment [7]. The determinants of higher rates of sudden death include severe symptoms and subnormal LVEF, but most sudden deaths occur in patients with no or minimal symptoms and normal LV function [7]. The rate of sudden death is 1.8% per year overall and even in patients without risk factors, is 0.8% per year. Therefore, the recent information on the natural history of MR underscores the serious prognostic implication of severe MR and suggests that surgery should be considered early in the course of the disease.

Progression of MR. The new quantitative techniques have allowed definition of the progression of MR. MR is a progressive disease [8], with an average increase of 7.5 ml/year in regurgitant volume and of 5.9 mm^2/year for the effective regurgitant orifice. The determinants of progression are anatomic changes, with more rapid progression in patients with MVP (particularly with development of new flail leaflet) and with enlarging mitral annulus [8]. Importantly, progression is not uniform. Half of patients manifest notable progression, but 11% evidence spontaneous regression of MR related to improved loading conditions. The progression of MR also causes progression of LV remodeling leading to LV dysfunction [9].

LV Dysfunction. How to assess LV function in MR is the subject of ongoing debate. The increased diastolic inflow volume increases preload. During systole, the regurgitant flow towards the left atrium suggests a decreased impedance

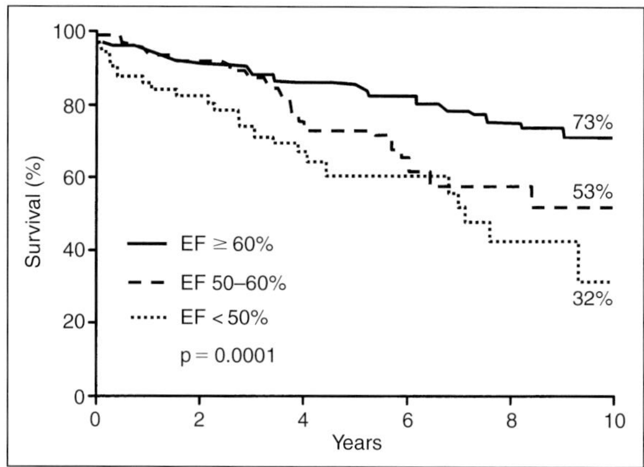

Fig. 2. Long-term post-operative survival according to the pre-operative echocardiographic EF. Note the excess mortality in patients with EF <50% but also with 'low normal' EF (50–59%) [from American Heart Association, Dallas, Tex., with permission].

to ejection, but end-systolic wall stress is usually normal. Multiple methods of correction of the measured LV function indices have been suggested, showing that there is no wide consensus on how to measure intrinsic LV function in MR.

Clinically, LV dysfunction is a major source of poor outcome under conservative management [6] or post-operatively [10]. Although currently, due to the progress of anesthesia and myocardial protection, peri-operative death is relatively uncommon, LV dysfunction is the most potent predictor of late death after surgery [10]. The LVEF decreases significantly, by approximately 10%, immediately after surgical correction of MR [9]. Therefore, despite symptomatic improvement, post-operative LV dysfunction (LVEF <50%) is frequent, occurring in close to one third of the patients successfully operated for organic MR. Post-operative LV dysfunction is associated with poor survival [9, 11] and high, but delayed, incidence of heart failure [12].

Pre-operative LVEF is the best predictor of long-term mortality under conservative management [6] and after surgery [10] (fig. 2), of congestive heart failure [12], and of post-operative residual LV function [9]. The end-systolic dimension is also a significant predictor of the post-operative LV function [9]. Therefore, either a LVEF <60% or an end-systolic diameter ⩾45 mm indicate overt LV dysfunction and should mandate immediate surgery in the absence of major comorbidities [13].

However, reduced LV function, even marked, should not be considered a contraindication to surgery in patients with organic MR because operative mortality is not excessive is these patients [10] and because the post-operative clinical complications are often delayed after surgery. Also, the precision of the prediction of outcome is imperfect, with a relatively wide range of error for the prediction of post-operative LV function [9, 11, 14]. As the best outcome is observed in patients with LVEF ⩾60%, this stage of the disease appears to represent the best opportunity for surgery. Therefore, the concept of waiting for signs of early decline of LV function is rigged with a notable risk of 'unexpected' LV dysfunction [9] and appears defensible mostly when the MR is not severe enough to warrant immediate surgery, the operative risk is high, or the chances of a valve repair are low.

Recent Progress of Mitral Surgery

In the early 1980s, the *operative mortality* was too high to consider surgery in asymptomatic patients. However, for patients with organic MR, operative mortality has decreased considerably [15] and currently, in our institution, is around 1% in patients ⩽75 years whether repair or replacement is performed [10]. Conversely, the operative mortality in patients ⩾75 years old, although improving recently, remains relatively high, between 3.5 and 12%, depending on the pre-operative presentation [16].

The development of *valve repair* has transformed clinical practice in MR [17]. In early reports [18–20], the lower operative mortality and better long-term survival after valve repair than replacement may have been due to a better pre-operative condition of patients undergoing valve repair or to the procedure itself. In our experience, taking into account all differences at baseline between valve repairs and replacements, valve repair is indeed an independent predictor of a better outcome after surgery for MR with a lower operative mortality and a better long-term survival than after valve replacement [3]. This benefit is noted whether or not associated coronary bypass surgery is performed [3]. A major reason for the improved outcome after valve repair is better LV function than after valve replacement [3]. The conservation of the subvalvular apparatus certainly plays a role in the preserved LV function after valve repair as it does after valve replacement without transsection of chordae. The improved survival after valve repair is not accomplished at the expense of an increased risk of reoperation [3]. Our most recent data looking at the very long-term outcome of valve repair compared to valve replacement shows that the benefit in term of survival is observed not only for posterior leaflet prolapse but also for anterior leaflet prolapse [21]. Therefore, irrespective of the localization of the prolapse, valve repair should be the preferred type of surgical correction of MR.

Intra-operative transesophageal echocardiography is an essential component of the success of valve repair and should be performed by experienced physicians to monitor the repair procedure and help with intra-operative decisions [22]. Therefore, valve repair has become extremely popular [23]. Currently, in 85–90% of patients with isolated MR, a successful repair can be performed. This high percentage of repair has been achievable (after the initial learning phase of this difficult procedure) through the utilization of special techniques such as the transposition of chordae or insertion of artificial chordae, the latter in particular for the rupture chords of the anterior leaflet [24, 25]. However, the reparability of rheumatic lesions is not as consistent as that of degenerative lesions [26]. Despite these high feasibility rates, the repair of the mitral valve should not be considered as a panacea and does not eliminate the risk of myocardial dysfunction. In patients with LVEF <60%, an excess mortality is noted whether repair or replacement is performed [3]. Therefore, the ability to perform repair in a high percentage of patients should be considered as an incentive to perform surgery because of its low risk and good survival and not as an incentive to delay surgery and encounter the risk of more LV dysfunction.

Outcome after Surgical Correction of Mitral Regurgitation

To make appropriate decisions, it is important to analyze the predictors of poor post-operative outcome.

LV dysfunction (defined as LVEF <60% and/or end-systolic diameter ⩾45 mm) imposes an excess rate of long-term mortality [10] and heart failure [12] compared to patients with better function at surgery.

Class III or IV symptoms before surgery are not benign. In our experience, the more severe the pre-operative symptoms were, the lower the post-operative LVEF [9] and the higher the incidence of post-operative congestive heart failure [12]. Adjusting for age at surgery and all other determinants of outcome, severe pre-operative symptoms are associated with worse long-term survival [16, 27] and excess incidence of heart failure [12]. Even in the privileged subgroup of patients with LVEF ⩾60%, in whom survival is not different from the expected survival, patients operated at an early stage with minimal symptoms have a better survival than patients with severe symptoms [10]. Therefore, waiting for severe symptoms is associated with a higher incidence of complications after the surgery is performed (fig. 3).

Atrial fibrillation (AF) persisting for more than 3 months before surgery is associated with a high risk of post-operative persistence of AF. Conversely, recent AF tends to revert to sinus rhythm post-operatively [28]. Therefore, waiting for chronic AF pre-operatively is associated with residual post-operative morbidity.

There is no randomized trial comparing the *outcome after early surgery* for organic MR to the outcome with medical management. However, in patients

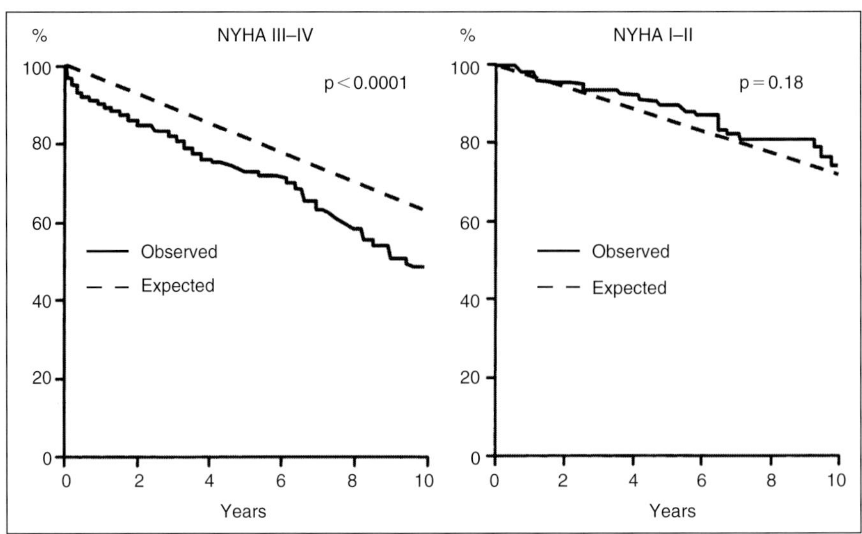

Fig. 3. Comparison of observed and expected survival after surgical correction of MR separately in patients pre-operatively with severe symptoms (left) and minimal or no symptoms (right). There is excess mortality in patients operated with severe symptoms but no excess mortality in patients who had no or minimal symptoms, suggesting that in the latter group the long-term consequences of MR have been suppressed [from American Heart Association, Dallas, Tex., with permission].

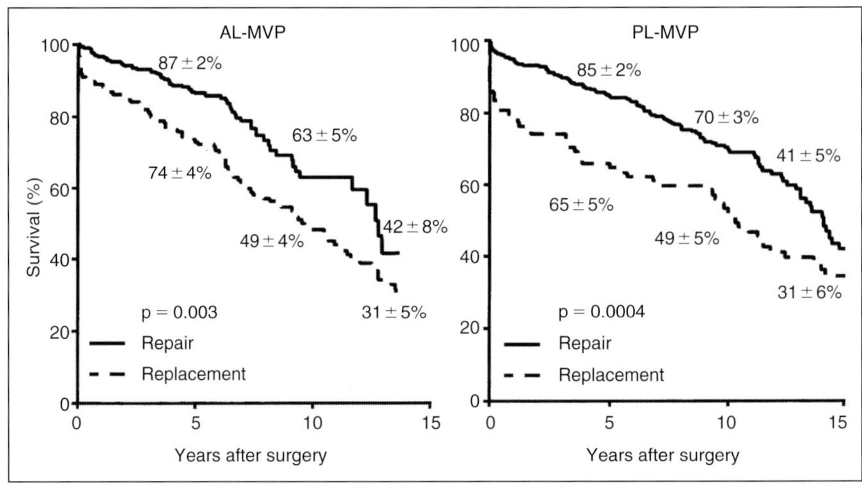

Fig. 4. Long-term survival after surgical correction of MR for MVP involving the anterior leaflet (left) or confined to the posterior leaflet (right). In both types of prolapse the survival is significantly better after valve repair than after valve replacement.

with flail mitral leaflets, the long-term outcome after early surgery was compared to that of patients managed conservatively and operated whenever it was judged necessary. Although many patients initially treated conservatively eventually underwent surgery, the early surgical approach was associated with an improved long-term survival through a marked reduction in cardiac mortality and decreased morbidity (less heart failure and less AF) during follow-up [29]. These results underline the potential for eliminating most of the cardiac complications due to MR through an early surgical approach as long as the operative mortality remains low (<2%).

Clinical Decision-Making in Mitral Regurgitation

It is important to gather appropriate information to define the timing of surgery.

Symptoms. The severity of symptoms is defined by history, but as many patients progressively limit their physical activity, performing exercise testing in 'asymptomatic' patients [30], in particular with oxygen consumption measurement, may unveil unexpected exercise limitations.

LV Function. LV function usually is assessed by echocardiography <60% or LV end-systolic diameter ⩾45 mm are considered signs of overt LV dysfunction.

Degree of MR Hemodynamics. Although the extent of the MR jet by color flow imaging or the density of dye in the left atrium by angiography are useful to quantify MR, these methods have numerous pitfalls [31, 32]. Comprehensive assessment of MR severity can be performed by quantitative Doppler echocardiography. The most widely used method of quantitation is the PISA method, based on the analysis of the flow convergence region proximal to the regurgitant orifice [33, 34]. The Doppler measurement of mitral and aortic stroke volumes is also useful but more cumbersome to master [35]. Both methods allow calculation of the regurgitant volume (RVol) and effective regurgitant orifice (ERO) [36]. The respective thresholds for severe MR are ⩾60 ml for RVol and ⩾40 mm^2 for ERO. Hemodynamics can also be characterized by measuring the cardiac output by Doppler and the right ventricular systolic pressure by use of the tricuspid regurgitant velocity.

Etiology-Repairability. The mitral lesions can be reliably characterized by echocardiography [37]. Usually, transthoracic echocardiography is sufficient but when imaging is mediocre, transesophageal echocardiography can be helpful [37]. Rheumatic lesions or massive calcifications of the valve or annulus often are difficult to repair but in the vast majority of cases, MVP is repairable. The reparability is highly dependent on the skills and experience of the surgeon and should be defined from both patient- and institution-based criteria. New methods have extended the field of application of repair, particularly with anterior leaflet flail segments [25], but if local experience is limited, it is important to refer patients to centers with more extensive experience.

Surgical Risk. The operative risk is mostly determined by age (high risk if ⩾75 years) [10], by the presence of severe pre-operative heart failure [16], by the presence of coronary disease [38], and by the severity of comorbid conditions. A composite assessment of the risk is essential for clinical decision-making, but the risk in asymptomatic patients ⩽75 years old is usually low, between 0.1 and 0.2% in most advanced centers.

The timing of surgical correction of MR is then based on the combination of these observations, and the decision is either prompt mitral surgery or rather follow-up with conservative management.

Severe MR with Overt Symptoms or LV Dysfunction. Patients with severe MR with overt severe consequences should be offered surgery even when risk is relatively high and irrespective of reparability of the mitral valve. Although surgery performed with this type of presentation results in symptomatic improvement, it is associated with notable excess post-operative risk [10, 16]. However, the post-operative outcome is far better than the outcome under medical treatment [6].

Severe MR with neither Overt Symptoms nor LV Dysfunction. Irrespective of reparability, some recent events before the visit are strong incentives to propose surgery immediately: AF, even if paroxysmal, ventricular tachycardia at rest or during exercise, or the observation of pulmonary hypertension by echocardiography are such findings [13]. With *low probability of repair*, patients are usually not referred to surgery if there are no clinical risk factors. However, patients with massive MR (RVol ⩾100 ml/beat) or with marked left atrial enlargement may be considered for surgery if they are at low surgical risk. With *high probability of valve repair*, our approach [29] and the current guidelines [13] have become much more aggressive towards surgery, even if there are no symptoms or signs of LV dysfunction, if the operative risk is low. This aggressive approach will require a randomized clinical trial in the future to define the magnitude of its benefit.

MR Not Severe. For RVols <45 ml/beat, there is almost never a need for surgery, and there is concern that a failed repair attempted during another cardiac operation (such as bypass surgery needed for angina) may result in worse MR than originally present. For RVols 45–60 ml/beat, there is usually no need for immediate surgery, but in certain rare circumstances mitral surgery may be indicated. These involve valves that are reparable and patients who need a cardiac operation for a maze procedure or coronary bypass surgery or another valve surgery. In some patients with MVP and ventricular tachycardia at rest or with exertion, we have performed a mitral valve repair to suppress the volume overload. The comparison of a surgical approach to medical treatment and even the determination of the benefit of medical treatment under those circumstances remains to be defined [13].

Conclusion

The timing of surgery for MR has changed considerably from a relatively passive response to the development of severe symptoms to an early surgery concept preceding the signs of LV dysfunction. Early surgery requires a high repair rate and a low operative mortality. Therefore, currently, not all patients and not all institutions are candidates to apply the early indications of surgical correction of MR. Nevertheless, considerable progress has recently been accomplished for the assessment and treatment of MR. Surgery should be considered early in the course of the disease, when severe MR has been identified.

References

1 Singh J, Evans J, Levy D, et al: Prevalence and clinical determinants of mitral, tricuspid and aortic regurgitation. Am J Cardiol 1999;83:897–902.
2 Olson L, Subramanian R, Ackermann D, Orszulak T, Edwards W: Surgical pathology of the mitral valve: A study of 712 cases spanning 21 years. Mayo Clin Proc 1987;62:22–34.
3 Enriquez-Sarano M, Schaff H, Orszulak T, Tajik A, Bailey K, Frye R: Valve repair improves the outcome of surgery for mitral regurgitation. Circulation 1995;91:1264–1265.
4 Delahaye J, Gare J, Viguier E, Delahaye F, De Gevigney G, Milon H: Natural history of severe mitral regurgitation. Eur Heart J 1991;12(suppl B):5–9.
5 Horstkotte D, Loogen F, Kleikamp G, Schulte H, Trampisch H, Bircks W: Effect of prosthetic heart valve replacement on the natural course of isolated mitral and aortic as well as multivalvular diseases. Clinical results in 783 patients up to 8 years following implantation of the Björk-Shiley tilting disc prosthesis. Z Kardiol 1983;72:494–503.
6 Ling H, Enriquez-Sarano M, Seward J, et al: Clinical outcome of mitral regurgitation due to flail leaflets. N Engl J Med 1996;335:1417–1423.
7 Grigioni F, Enriquez-Sarano M, Ling L, et al: Sudden death in mitral regurgitation due to flail leaflet. J Am Coll Cardiol 1999;34:2078–2085.
8 Enriquez-Sarano M, Basmadjian A, Rossi A, Bailey K, Seward J, Tajik A: Progression of mitral regurgitation: A prospective Doppler echocardiographic study. J Am Coll Cardiol 1999;34: 1137–1144.
9 Enriquez-Sarano M, Tajik A, Schaff H, et al: Echocardiographic prediction of left ventricular function after correction of mitral regurgitation: Results and clinical implications. J Am Coll Cardiol 1994;24:1536–1543.
10 Enriquez-Sarano M, Tajik A, Schaff H, Orszulak T, Bailey K, Frye R: Echocardiographic prediction of survival after surgical correction of organic mitral regurgitation. Circulation 1994;90: 830–837.
11 Crawford M, Souchek J, Oprian C, et al: Determinants of survival and left ventricular performance after mitral valve replacement. Circulation 1990;81:1173–1181.
12 Enriquez-Sarano M, Schaff H, Orszulak T, Bailey K, Tajik A, Frye R: Congestive heart failure after surgical correction of mitral regurgitation. A long-term study. Circulation 1995;92:2496–2503.

13 Bonow R, Carabello B, DeLeon A, et al: ACC/AHA guidelines for the management of patients with valvular heart disease. Circulation 1998;98:1949–1984.

14 Leung D, Griffin B, Stewart W, Cosgrove D, Thomas J, Marwick T: Left ventricular function after valve repair for chronic mitral regurgitation: Predictive value of preoperative assessment of contractile reserve by exercise echocardiography. J Am Coll Cardiol 1996;28:1198–1205.

15 Cohn L, Couper G, Kinchla N, Collins JJ: Decreased operative risk of surgical treatment of mitral regurgitation with or without coronary artery disease. J Am Coll Cardiol 1990;16:1575–1578.

16 Tribouilloy C, Enriquez-Sarano M, Schaff H, et al: Impact of preoperative symptoms on survival after surgical correction of organic mitral regurgitation: Rationale for optimizing surgical indications. Circulation 1999;99:400–405.

17 Carpentier A: Cardiac valve surgery – The 'French Correction'. J Thorac Cardiovasc Surg 1983; 86:323–337.

18 Cohn L, Kowalker W, Bhatia S, et al: Comparative morbidity of mitral valve repair versus replacement for mitral regurgitation with and without coronary artery disease. Ann Thorac Surg 1988;45: 284–290.

19 Perier P, Deloche A, Chauvaud S, et al: Comparative evaluation of mitral valve repair and replacement with Starr, Bjork and porcine valve prostheses. Circulation 1984;70:187–192.

20 Sand M, Naftel D, Blackstone E, Kirklin J, Karp R: A comparison of repair and replacement for mitral valve incompetence. J Thorac Cardiovasc Surg 1987;94:208–219.

21 Mohty D, Orszulak TA, Schaff HV, Avierinos JF, Tajik JA, Enriquez-Sarano M: Very long-term survival and durability of mitral valve repair for mitral valve prolapse. Circulation 2001;104 (suppl 1):1–I7.

22 Freeman W, Schaff H, Khanderia B, et al: Intraoperative evaluation of mitral valve regurgitation and repair by transesophageal echocardiography: Incidence and significance of systolic anterior motion. J Am Coll Cardiol 1992;20:599–609.

23 Cosgrove D, Chavez A, Lytle B, et al: Results of mitral valve reconstruction. Circulation 1986;74: 82–87.

24 Frater R, Gabbay S, Shore D, Factor S, Strom J: Reproducible replacement of elongated or ruptured mitral valve chordae. Ann Thorac Surg 1983;35:14–28.

25 Lessana A, Escorsin M, Romano M, et al: Transposition of posterior leaflet for treatment of ruptured main chordae of the anterior mitral leaflet. J Thorac Cardiovasc Surg 1985;89:804–806.

26 Gillinov A, Cosgrove D, Blackstone E, et al: Durability of mitral valve repair for degenerative disease. J Thorac Cardiovasc Surg 1998;116:734–743.

27 Sousa Uva M, Dreyfus G, Rescigno G, et al: Surgical treatment of asymptomatic and mildly symptomatic mitral regurgitation. J Thorac Cardiovasc Surg 1996;112:1240–1249.

28 Chua Y, Schaff H, Orszulak T, Morriss J: Outcome of mitral valve repair in patients with preoperative atrial fibrillation. Should the maze procedure be combined with mitral valvuloplasty? J Thorac Cardiovasc Surg 1994;107:408–415.

29 Ling L, Enriquez-Sarano M, Seward J, et al: Early surgery in patients with mitral regurgitation due to partial flail leaflet: A long-term outcome study. Circulation 1997;96:1819–1825.

30 Leung D, Griffin B, Snader C, Luthern L, Thomas JD, Marwick T: Determinants of functional capacity in chronic mitral regurgitation unassociated with coronary artery disease or left ventricular dysfunction. Am J Cardiol 1997;79:914–920.

31 Enriquez-Sarano M, Tajik A, Bailey K, Seward J: Color flow imaging compared with quantitative Doppler assessment of severity of mitral regurgitation: Influence of eccentricity of jet and mechanism of regurgitation. J Am Coll Cardiol 1993;21:1211–1219.

32 Croft C, Lipscomb K, Mathis K, et al: Limitations of qualitative angiographic grading in aortic or mitral regurgitation. Am J Cardiol 1984;53:1593–1598.

33 Enriquez-Sarano M, Miller FJ, Hayes S, Bailey K, Tajik A, Seward J: Effective mitral regurgitant orifice area: Clinical use and pitfalls of the proximal isovelocity surface area method. J Am Coll Cardiol 1995;25:703–709.

34 Vandervoort P, Rivera J, Mele D, et al: Application of color Doppler flow mapping to calculate effective regurgitant orifice area. An in vitro study and initial clinical observations. Circulation 1993;88:1150–1156.

35 Enriquez-Sarano M, Bailey K, Seward J, Tajik A, Krohn M, Mays J: Quantitative Doppler assessment of valvular regurgitation. Circulation 1993;87:841–848.
36 Enriquez-Sarano M, Seward J, Bailey K, Tajik A: Effective regurgitant orifice area: A noninvasive Doppler development of an old hemodynamic concept. J Am Coll Cardiol 1994;23:443–451.
37 Enriquez-Sarano M, Freeman W, Tribouilloy C, et al: Functional anatomy of mitral regurgitation: Echocardiographic assessment and implications on outcome. J Am Coll Cardiol 1999;34:1129–1136.
38 Tribouilloy C, Enriquez-Sarano M, Schaff H, et al: Excess mortality due to coronary artery disease after valvular surgery: Secular trends in valvular regurgitation and effect of internal mammary bypass. Circulation 1998;98(suppl):108–115.

Dr. Maurice Enriquez-Sarano, Mayo Clinic, 200 First Street SW,
Rochester, MN 55905 (USA)

Borer JS, Isom OW (eds): Pathophysiology, Evaluation and Management of Valvular Heart Diseases.
Adv Cardiol. Basel, Karger, 2002, vol 39, pp 144–152

Importance of Right Ventricular Performance Measurement in Selecting Asymptomatic Patients with Mitral Regurgitation for Valve Surgery

Jeffrey S. Borer, Clare A. Hochreiter, Phyllis G. Supino, Edmund McM. Herrold, Karl H. Krieger, O. Wayne Isom

Division of Cardiovascular Pathophysiology, Department of Cardiothoracic Surgery and The Howard Gilman Institute for Valvular Heart Diseases, Weill Medical College of Cornell University, New York, N.Y., USA

The asymptomatic patient with mitral regurgitation (MR) can present a difficult management dilemma. As long as left ventricular ejection fraction (LVEF) is well within normal limits (>10% above the lower limit of normal [usually >60%] from the data of Enriquez-Sarano et al. [1]), survival after mitral valve surgery is not significantly different from that expected in the age-matched US population irrespective of disease. When LV performance falls below this standard, or if symptoms develop (even if LVEF is well maintained), late post-operative survival deteriorates. Given the relatively low risk now associated with mitral valve repair procedures, the late post-operative burden caused by even relatively mild pre-operative LV dysfunction or symptoms has led to the generally accepted suggestion that 'prophylactic' mitral valve repair should be performed in asymptomatic patients with LVEF <60%. Many in the field have gone further, however, suggesting that this surgical procedure should be offered to anyone with severe MR, irrespective of the status of LVEF. This more aggressive suggestion is based, first, on a lack of consensus that currently available evaluation strategies can predict imminent development of symptoms or LVEF <60% and, second, on the relatively low risk of mitral valve repair, the belief that the current version of this operation virtually restores physiological valve function (or does so as well as is likely to be possible) and that, therefore, there is no advantage to delay that could allow prognostically important myocardial dysfunction to develop.

Also, this suggestion presupposes that (a) the risk of operation truly is trivial and, in any event, is no higher than the risk of not operating in an asymptomatic patient with well-maintained LVEF, (b) all patients who enter the operating room for a mitral valve repair do, in fact, undergo repair rather than replacement (which carries higher risk and added long-term problems), i.e., no technical factors that were unsuspected before operation can preclude a planned repair and (c) the repair is the most appropriate procedure for all patients with MR for whom it is technically possible, i.e., no anatomical or other factors can mitigate short- or long-term benefit from this approach. It is not clear that these latter presuppositions truly are legitimate; thus, it is not clear that all patients with MR should undergo repair merely because the valve lesion is severe. The problem, then, is identification of patients for whom clinical deterioration, with concomitant worsening of long-term prognosis, can be confidently predicted despite absence of symptoms and well-maintained LVEF at rest.

The low impedence outflow pathway into the left atrium that helps to preserve LVEF in patients with MR simultaneously serves to impede right ventricular (RV) outflow, potentially impacting on the long-term status of the RV myocardium. This fact suggests an approach to resolving the problem of predicting patients at risk, based on assessment of RV performance.

Although modern statistical assessments often were not performed, review of early cardiac surgical literature leads to the strong inference that severity of pulmonary hypertension measured before operation is a primary determinant of early and long-term post-operative survival after mitral valve replacement for MR [2, 3]. Pulmonary artery pressure also is a primary determinant of RVEF [4]. Therefore, we hypothesized that measurement of RVEF modifies prognostication based on LVEF alone, and may be useful in identifying the asymptomatic patient for operation.

Development and Application of RVEF Measurement for MR

In 1971, an elderly woman was admitted to the then National Heart and Lung Institute with severe mitral valve disease (MR and mitral stenosis). Though LVEF was reasonably well preserved, she had moderately severe pulmonary hypertension. She underwent mitral valve replacement and returned after 6 months for recatheterization (standard procedure at the National Institutes of Health in that era). Her pulmonary hypertension had improved, but she was troubled by severe fatigue and persistent right heart failure, despite a technically successful operation, and died relatively shortly thereafter. Though a measure of RVEF was not readily available at the time, hemodynamic and functional evaluation suggested that the most severe and irreversible myocardial damage resided in the RV and that this was the predominant cause of the poor outcome. The lack of an easily applied measure of RVEF resulted primarily from the fact that the RV is geometrically irregular, limiting the accuracy of volume determination from geometric formulae applied to dimensional data. The difficulty with geometric calculation is greatest when data are obtained in a single plane, the standard for contrast angiography and echocardiography at the time but, in fact, also adversely affects results when data are available in several planes. In 1976, when we developed equilibrium radionuclide cineangiography, a geometry-independent method finally was available [5]; soon, this tool was applied for RVEF determination [6, 7], and then to resolution of risk assessment in patients with MR [4, 8–11]. The methodology of RVEF determination with radionuclide angiography differs depending on whether first-pass (the standard for RVEF evaluation) or equilibrium techniques are employed. Most data relative to prognostication have been produced with the equilibrium method. This involves intravenous administration of a radioactive tracer in a form in which it will remain in the intravascular space throughout the period of imaging; the tracer is allowed to mix thoroughly within the intravascular space so that placement of a radiation detector over the patient's chest and collection of radioactive emissions will result in data that define the relative magnitude of the subjacent blood volume. Emissions that are identified by the detector are transmitted in electronic format to a computer, which displays the data as a series of highly temporally resolved single-plane images, or frames. The images are divided into picture elements (pixels) that allow computer-based determination of regional distribution of the radioactive emissions. Identification of the RV outline, defining a 'region of interest' (ROI), is performed in the end-diastolic frame, collected during an interval of $\leqslant$40 ms immediately following the ECG QRS complex. Similar images from many successive cardiac cycles (total collection time $\geqslant$2 min) are superimposed to provide the final image from which count density in the RV ROI can be defined. A background region, usually adjacent to the LV, then is selected, average counts per background pixel is calculated and the average background is subtracted from each pixel in the end-diastolic and end-systolic RV ROIs. The resulting background-subtracted values are directly proportional to RV end-diastolic and end-systolic volumes, enabling calculation of RVEF [6, 7]. This procedure has been validated by comparison both with contrast angiography by digital, non-geometric methods, and with first-pass radionuclide angiographic determinations [6, 7]. As previously noted, RVEF is inversely related to pulmonary artery pressure both in patients with MR and with other causes of pulmonary hypertension. Since symptoms result from pulmonary vascular congestion, it is not surprising that, with MR, RVEF during exercise is directly related to exercise tolerance, an objectification of symptoms (fig. 1); the relation between LVEF during exercise and exercise tolerance is poor to non-existent in MR [4]. Thus, RVEF, but not LVEF, has a clear relation

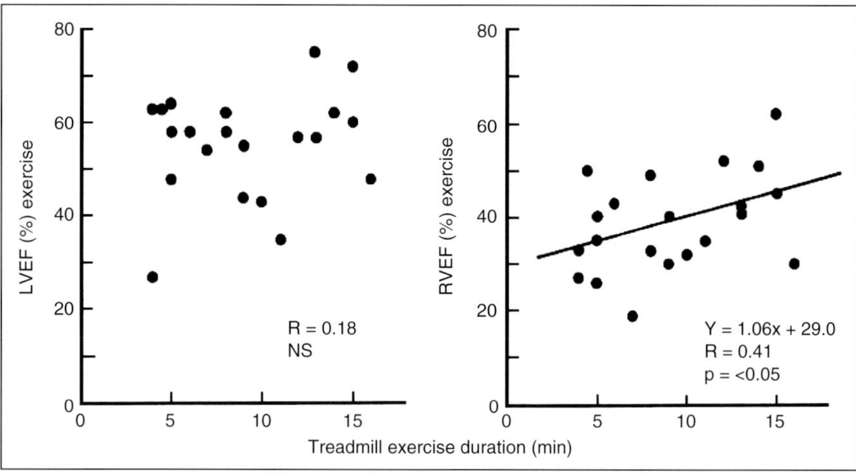

Fig. 1. Exercise tolerance as function of RVEF and LVEF during exercise, from the first 42 patients of the subsequently published report of EF in prognostication [4], as initially presented; while the final (53-patient) enlarged series showed a very modest but significant relation of exercise tolerance and $LVEF_{exercise}$ (never published in graphic form), a far stronger and significant relation was apparent when $RVEF_{exercise}$ was evaluated.

to clinical debility in this disease. Pre-operative RVEF also is a primary determinant of symptom status *after* mitral valve surgery, even though pulmonary hypertension largely has been resolved [12]; in the late post-operative setting, LV contractility is a better predictor of symptom status, but the persistent predictive value of RVEF after resolution of major hemodynamic abnormalities indicates the importance of the RV myocardium in the pathophysiology of MR [12].

Prognostication Using RVEF

In an early study involving 53 patients with MR, among whom 32 were unoperated and 21 had undergone mitral valve surgery, RVEF was strongly predictive of outcome in the unoperated group [4]. When RVEF was subnormal (<35%) at the index study, mortality was almost 50% during an average 2.3-year follow-up. However, this result was heavily influenced by the outcome among patients in whom RVEF was moderately subnormal, that is, ≤30%: for these patients, mortality exceeded 80% during the relatively short follow-up. Indeed, all deaths in this group occurred within 2 years of study initiation, and most were sudden and presumably arrhythmic, rather than secondary to pump dysfunction and intractable heart failure. No patient died during the initial 2.3 years of follow-up if RVEF was >30% (fig. 2). Though the small size of the

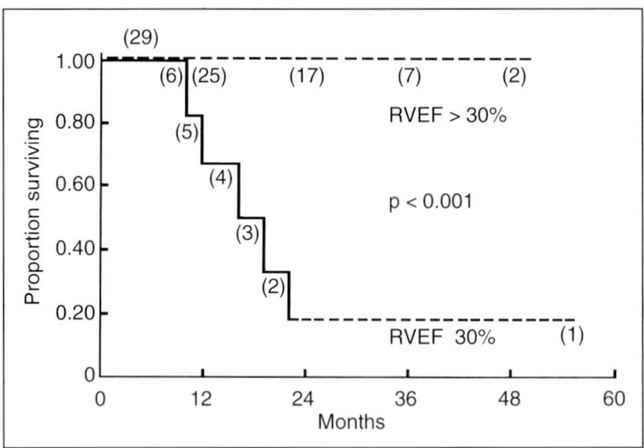

Fig. 2. Survival among patients with hemodynamically severe MR as a function of RVEF at rest [from 4, with permission].

series precludes the inference that this mortality point estimate is statistically stable, the results nonetheless confirm the potency of RVEF as a prognosticator in MR. Moreover, while subnormal LVEF also indicated particularly poor prognosis, RVEF was the more powerful and independent predictor.

From these data it is clear that by the time RVEF is subnormal at rest, prognosis is importantly compromised. Prediction of the imminence of this development, or of less dire 'high-risk descriptors', requires a different measure. In several heart diseases, LV dysfunction can be unmasked by exercise, carrying prognostically useful information, at a midway point between totally normal function and dysfunction apparent at rest [13, 14]. Similarly, interrogation of RV function during exercise should provide prognostically useful insights in MR. This likelihood was suggested empirically by the finding that, in patients with combined severe MR and severe aortic regurgitation, exercise-induced RV dysfunction was the single best predictor of late post-operative mortality [10]. Subsequently, in a study of 44 asymptomatic patients with MR and with normal LVEF and RVEF at rest, we found that progression to symptomatic heart failure was predicted best by the change (Δ) in RVEF from rest to exercise. Thus, for the entire cohort, heart failure occurred at a rate of approximately 10% per year. However, the study population could be dichotomized into a subgroup with a progression rate of approximately 14% per year and another that progressed at a rate of less than 4% per year based on the response of RVEF to exercise. If RVEF increased during exercise, progression was relatively slow. If RVEF did not increase during exercise, progression to heart failure was more rapid. Moreover, in the preliminary analysis of these data, progression to subnormal ventricular performance occasionally, though rarely, preceded symptom development [15]. When the final report of this study was published, only the 31-patient ‘etiologically pure’ subcohort with MR due to mitral valve prolapse was assessed, and revealed progression rates similar to those for the group as a whole [9]. These data indicate that the risk of heart failure is almost 50% over 3 years for patients who are asymptomatic with well-preserved LVEF and RVEF at rest but who demonstrate compromised RV functional reserve, while the risk of such progression is substantially less for those with initially well-preserved RV functional reserve. (Relative risk is 3- to 5-fold greater for those with negative ΔRVEF when the entire series, mitral valve prolapse alone and with other non-ischemic etiologies, is considered.) Indeed, RVEF response to exercise was the only predictor of progression; neither LVEF (rest or exercise or ΔLVEF from rest to exercise) nor any echocardiographic measure demonstrated predictive value in this group [9].

While RV dysfunction indicates important risk to life in the absence of valve surgery, mitral valve replacement or repair improves survival significantly among patients who manifest high-risk RV descriptors. In our initial series, among patients with RVEF ≤30% at rest, only 17% survived during an average 2.3-year follow-up, irrespective of LVEF, while 83% survived during an average 2.5-year follow-up among those who underwent surgery ($p < 0.05$) [4]. When this series was enlarged and lengthened to enable determination of the predictors of late post-operative survival, the earlier findings were confirmed and strengthened and, again, RVEF was the predominant predictive variable [11]. Thus, in a study of 23 patients with subnormal LVEF and/or RVEF ≤30% at rest, 14 underwent mitral valve surgery and were followed an average of 9 years after operation. Survival in the surgical cohort averaged 12.6 years and was significantly ($p = 0.0001$) better than that of the unoperated comparators, whose average survival was 3.8 years. This result was maintained ($p < 0.0001$) even when patients were rigorously matched for pre-operative LVEF to avoid possible effects of unintentional bias due to referrals away from operation of patients with severe LV dysfunction. However, among the surgical cohort, survival was significantly tied to pre-operative RVEF: though the number of events was too small to establish stable point estimates, deaths occurred earlier and more frequently among those with RVEF ≤20% at rest (fig. 3). Thus, survival after operation averaged 6.9 years for those with RVEF ≤20% at rest and 14 years for those whose RVEF exceeded 20% ($p = 0.032$). Dichotomization of the surgical population was similar when RVEF during exercise was used as the discriminator.

Conclusions

Asymptomatic patients with severe MR and LVEF >60% manifest excellent survival after mitral valve surgery. Indeed, survival in this group equals that

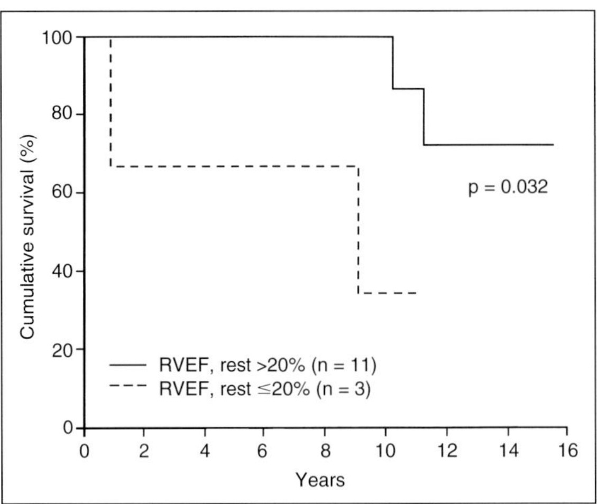

Fig. 3. Survival late after mitral valve surgery as a function of RVEF at rest among patients with severe MR and subnormal left and or RVEF before operation [from 11, with permission].

of an age-matched reference population. Symptoms enhance risk, even if LVEF is well maintained before operation. Symptoms result from pulmonary vascular congestion which, in turn, ultimately causes RV dysfunction. RVEF is a direct measure of the impact on the myocardium of the pulmonary hypertension that results secondarily from pulmonary vascular congestion in MR. When RVEF is subnormal at rest, even without symptoms, mortality risk is quite high unless operation is performed. Mitral valve surgery is life-prolonging in such patients, and should be performed as soon as possible. However, loss of RV functional reserve, that is, a fall in RVEF during exercise compared with the resting value, often is seen in the absence of symptoms, when LVEF is >60% and RVEF is normal at rest. This finding identifies a patient with almost a 50% likelihood of developing heart failure during the next 3 years in the absence of surgery. Thus, RV dysfunction unmasked by exercise provides relatively early evidence of prognostically important myocardial alteration secondary to MR, earlier than all other descriptors commonly used today to identify patients for whom 'prophylactic' mitral valve surgery is appropriate. It seems intuitively reasonable, pending empirical or epidemiological evidence to the contrary, that this finding should be sought before deciding to operate in an asymptomatic patient with severe MR and well-preserved LV performance. Indeed, it seems reasonable to withhold operation from asymptomatic patients with well-preserved (>60%) LVEF at rest, normal RVEF at rest and RVEF that increases from rest to exercise until RV functional reserve deteriorates. Thus, decisions to operate in asymptomatic patients may be beneficially modifiable by evaluation of the RVEF.

Acknowledgements

Dr. Borer is the Gladys and Roland Harriman Professor of Cardiovascular Medicine at Cornell and was supported in part during this work by an endowment from the Gladys and Roland Harriman Foundation, New York, N.Y. In addition, the work reported herein was supported in part by National Heart Lung and Blood Institute, Bethesda, Md. (RO1- HL-26504), and by grants from The Howard Gilman Foundation, New York, N.Y., The Schiavone Family Foundation, White House Station, N.J., The Charles and Jean Brunie Foundation, Bronxville, N.Y., The David Margolis Foundation, New York, N.Y., The American Cardio-Vascular Research Foundation, New York, N.Y., The Irving R. Hansen Foundation, New York, N.Y., The Mary A.H. Rumsey Foundation, New York, N.Y., The Messinger Family Foundation, New York, N.Y., the Daniel and Elaine Sargent Charitable Trust, New York, N.Y., the A.C. Israel Foundation, Greenwich, Conn., and by much appreciated gifts from Maryjane and the late William Voute, Bronxville, N.Y., and Stephen and Suzanne Weiss, Greenwich, Conn.

References

1 Enriquez-Sarano M, Tajik AJ, Schaff HV, Orszulak TA, Bailey KR, Frye RL: Echocardiographic prediction of survival after surgical correction of organic mitral regurgitation. Circulation 1994;90:830–837.

2 Salomon NW, Stinson EB, Griepp RB, Shumway NE: Patient-related risk factors as predictors of results following isolated mitral valve replacement. Ann Thorac Surg 1977;24:519–530.

3 Morrow AG, Oldham HN, Elkins RC, Braunwald E: Prosthetic replacement of the mitral valve: Pre-operative and post-operative clinical and hemodynamic assessments in 100 patients. Circulation 1967;35:962–979.

4 Hochreiter C, Niles N, Devereux RB, Kligfield P, Borer JS: Mitral regurgitation: Relationship of noninvasive descriptors of right and left ventricular performance to clinical and hemodynamic findings and to prognosis in medically and surgically treated patients. Circulation 1986;73:900–912.

5 Borer JS, Bacharach SL, Green MV, Kent KM, Epstein SE, Johnston GS: Real-time radionuclide cineangiography in the noninvasive evaluation of global and regional left ventricular function at rest and during exercise in patients with coronary artery disease. N Engl J Med 1977;296:839–844.

6 Maddahi J, Berman DS, Matsuoka DT, Waxman AD, Stankus KE, Forrester JS, Swan HJC: A new technique for assessing right ventricular ejection fraction using rapid multiple-gated equilibrium cardiac blood pool scintigraphy. Circulation 1979;60:581–589.

7 Goldberg HL, Herrold EM, Hochreiter C, Moses JW, Fisher J, Tamari I, Borer JS: Videodensitometric determination of right ventricular and left ventricular ejection fraction. Am J Noninvas Cardiol 1987;1:18–23.

8 Furer J, Hochreiter C, Niles NW, Devereux RB, Kligfield P, Pazer D, Sato N, Borer JS: Prediction of symptom status following mitral valve replacement for mitral regurgitation by preoperative echocardiographic measurement of the end-systolic stress to end-systolic volume ratio. Am J Noninvas Cardiol 1987;1:321–328.

9 Rosen S, Borer JS, Hochreiter C, Supino P, Roman M, Devereux RB, Kligfield P: Natural history of the asymptomatic/minimally symptomatic patient with normal right and left ventricular performance and severe mitral regurgitation due to mitral valve prolapse. Am J Cardiol 1994;74: 374–380.

10 Niles N, Borer JS, Kamen M, Hochreiter C, Devereux RB, Kligfield P: Pre-operative left and right ventricular performance in combined aortic and mitral regurgitation and comparison with isolated aortic or mitral regurgitation. Am J Cardiol 1990;65:1372–1378.
11 Wencker D, Borer JS, Hochreiter C, Devereux RB, Roman MJ, Kligfield P, Supino P, Krieger K, Isom OW: Preoperative predictors of late postoperative outcome among patients with non-ischemic mitral regurgitation with 'high risk' descriptors, and comparison with unoperated patients. Cardiology 2000;93:37–42.
12 Furer J, Hochreiter C, Niles NW, Devereux RB, Kligfield P, Pazer D, Sato N, Borer JS: Prediction of symptom status following mitral valve replacement for mitral regurgitation by preoperative echocardiographic measurement of the end-systolic stress to end-systolic volume ratio. Am J Noninvas Cardiol 1987;1:321–328.
13 Borer JS: Measurement of ventricular function and volume; in Zaret B, Beller G (eds): Nuclear Cardiology: State of the Art and Future Directions, ed 2. St Louis, Mosby, 1998, pp 201–215.
14 Borer JS, Supino PG: Radionuclide angiography. II. Equilibrium imaging; in Iskandrian A, Verani M (eds): Nuclear Cardiac Imaging: Principles and Applications, ed 3. Oxford, New York, 2002.
15 Rosen S, Borer JS, Hochreiter C, Roman M, Bucek J, Devereux R, Kligfield P: Natural history of asymptomatic severe mitral regurgitation: Dissociation of symptom development and ventricular performance? J Am Coll Cardiol 1990;15:236A.

Jeffrey S. Borer, MD, Division of Cardiovascular Pathophysiology,
The New York-Presbyterian Hospital, New York Weill Cornell Center,
525 East 68th Street, New York, NY 10021 (USA)

Borer JS, Isom OW (eds): Pathophysiology, Evaluation and Management of Valvular Heart Diseases.
Adv Cardiol. Basel, Karger, 2002, vol 39, pp 153–156

Mitral Valve Repair for Ischemic Mitral Regurgitation

Lawrence H. Cohn

Division of Cardiac Surgery, Brigham and Women's Hospital, Boston, Mass., USA

Mitral valve repair for ischemic mitral regurgitation (MR) is one of the most controversial topics in valve surgery at the present time [1–3]. Elsewhere in this volume are data regarding feasibility, relative ease, superb results and improved physiology after repair of the mitral valve when it, alone, is diseased. Ischemic MR is a little more complicated because the patients have two diseases: coronary artery disease and MR.

I am going to give you some reasons why one should almost always repair the mitral valve for ischemic MR. First, uncorrected chronic MR with coronary artery disease leads to decreased long-term survival [4]. In our study of 2,000 patients who underwent coronary bypass alone, uncorrected MR almost doubled the risk of late death. The vast majority of patients with ischemic MR require only an annuloplasty ring because of annular dilatation of the left ventricle. It is very unusual that a valve replacement operation is necessary in patients with ischemic MR.

I use the Cosgrove ring C band because the anterior leaflet is usually fixed at the aortic trigone, stitches are not needed there as they would be with an encircling ring. Although, there is considerable debate about this point [5], this makes the repair a 10- to 15-min operation. Since the problem is primarily annular dilatation, one downsize the ring in ischemic MR as one might upsize the ring in the floppy prolapsed valve.

Another surgical alternative, which is even quicker, is the Alfieri stitch, which results in a two-orifice mitral valve [6]. I favor not using this as an isolated procedure because there have been recurrences of MR when the stitch was pulled out. What we have done, however, is to use this stitch in conjunction with a ring, particularly in those patients who have very severe ischemic cardiomyopathy. Many cardiologists point to experience with such patients who do quite well for a limited period, perhaps up to 2 years, after which MR may recur. In these patients, as the left ventricle dilates, the papillary muscles are dragged downward and the leaflets are opened so MR recurs despite the initial stabilization by the ring. In some severe ischemic cardiomyopathic patients, we do the annuloplasty ring and the Alfieri stitch to prevent the late opening of the mitral valve due to the dilatation of the ventricle.

Of course, any focal structural abnormality associated with moderate MR during coronary artery bypass grafting (CABG) should be corrected. We resect the segment with a ruptured chord and advance the two leaflet sections toward each other using monofilament running sutures all the way so you have very little in the way of knots to promote any thromboembolic event. The vast majority of patients with ischemic MR require only a ring and perhaps this Alfieri stitch, which does not add much to the operation.

Conversely, if one does not do valve repair at CABG, the morbidity and mortality for reoperation, mitral valve repair or replacement with multiple patent coronary bypass grafts can be quite high, complicated and dangerous for the patient [7]. Patients referred with prior CABG and patent grafts, including the mammary artery bypass graft, who had 2+ MR at the time of the original operation, present with 4+ mitral MR, a big ventricle and heart failure. The operative risk in these patients can be formidable, particularly with a resternotomy [6]. In this situation, we have chosen to use a right thoracotomy, hypothermic low flow perfusion and a modified mitral valve incision via the right thoracotomy, reducing the mortality by avoiding the sternum [7]. Nevertheless, it is still a difficult operation for patients who have had a previous CABG and now require mitral valve surgery. It has been said that mitral valve repair surgery is preferable to replacement because of the preservation of left ventricular shape and function. This is primarily due to preservation of the papillary muscles and the chordae tendineae. There was a concept propagated about 30 years ago that if one cuts off the 'pop-off valve' during mitral valve replacement, it would increase the wall tension and cause the left ventricle to fall apart [8]. The truth was that surgeons in those days were cutting all the chordae tips of the papillary muscles nice and neat, a perfect operation, but in doing so they changed the elliptical shape of the ventricle from a football to a basketball.

Surgeons and cardiologists are often confused about the changing degree of MR at the time of surgery. Preoperatively, patients may have 2+ to 3+ MR, but in the operating room the MR goes away because general anesthesia unloads the ventricle by afterload reduction. When afterload is increased by increasing mean arterial pressure to ⩾80 mm Hg, the MR returns [9]. Therefore, the decision to repair should be made preoperatively so as not to be tempted by wishful thinking at the time of the operation. In a Brigham series of downgraded MR in 60 patients, one surgeon made a concentrated effort not to repair the valve.

After successful revascularization, 20/60 patients still had 3+ MR postoperatively, while only 14/60 had 1+ MR. The rest continued to have 2+ MR. This MR gets downgraded by transesophageal echocardiogram during operation, but it comes back postoperatively in a lot of patients if not repaired. It is also very hard to predict if MR is going to be relieved with just coronary bypass, particularly if congestive symptoms have been present. With congestive symptoms preoperatively, you have fixed MR, particularly with a decreased ejection fraction. In the patient with a borderline ejection fraction, a mitral valve repair should be done to avoid a worse outcome if one does not correct the MR. If the repair is not performed, it is likely that this patient will come back 2 years later with massive MR, a borderline ejection fraction and a relatively high risk at reoperation.

Chen et al. [10] looked at patients with MR and a left ventricular ejection fraction under 0.30 who had mitral valve repair and concomitant CABG. Their ejection fractions improved significantly, and they had a markedly improved long-term survival compared to similar people without mitral valve repair. On the other hand, acute, intermittent MR, sometimes associated with flash pulmonary edema, observed with ischemia does not need surgical attention and will get better when ones does a good coronary bypass operation.

In a frequently quoted paper late results were presented that suggested that ischemic MR does not require correction in most people [11]. This is a study based on data from the late 1970s early 1980s, when intraoperative transesophageal echocardiography was not a routine procedure. Transesophageal echocardiography is used in every single patient during valve surgery in our hospital and is one of the most valuable tools to evaluate ischemic MR.

Finally, there is marked improvement in the results of mitral valve repair with CABG due to improved myocardial protection techniques, perfusion and familiarity with the disease. The operative mortality at the Brigham and Women's Hospital is $<4\%$ for patients with ischemic MR undergoing concomitant bypass and mitral valve annuloplasty, down from 14% several years ago, a quite significant reduction [12].

Because of the data presented above, we are aggressive in our approach that moderate MR in the symptomatic patient with a reduced ejection fraction should be corrected by mitral valve repair with an annuloplasty ring, concomitantly with CABG.

References

1 Dion R: Ischemic mitral regurgitation: When and how should it be corrected? J Heart Valve Dis 1993;2:535–543.

2 Christenson JT, Simonet F, Bloch A, Maurice J, Velebit V, Schmuziger M: Should a mild to moderate ischemic mitral valve regurgitation in patients with poor left ventricular function be repaired or not? J Heart Valve Dis 1995;4:484–489.

3 Von Oppell UO, Stemmet F, Brink J, Commerford PJ, Heijke SAM: Ischemic mitral valve repair surgery. J Heart Valve Dis 2000;9:64–74.
4 Adler DS, Goldman L, O'Neil A, Cook EF, Mudge GH Jr, Shemin RJ, DiSesa VJ, Cohn LH, Collins JJ Jr: Long-term survival of more than 2,000 patients after coronary artery bypass grafting. Am J Cardiol 1986;58:195–202.
5 Timek T, Glasson JR, Dagum P, Green GR, Nistal JF, Komeda M, Daughters GT, Bolger AF, Foppiano LE, Ingels NB, Miller DC: Ring annuloplasty prevents delayed leaflet coaptation and mitral regurgitation during acute left ventricular ischemia. J Thorac Cardiovasc Surg 2000;119: 774–783.
6 Umana JP, Salehizadeh B, Derose JJ, Nahar T, Lotvin A, Shunichi H, Oz MC: 'Bow-tie' mitral valve repair: An adjuvant technique for ischemic mitral regurgitation. Ann Thorac Surg 1998;66: 1640–1646.
7 Byrne JG, Aranki SF, Adams DH, Rizzo RJ, Couper GS, Cohn LH: Mitral valve surgery after previous CABG with functioning IMA grafts. Ann Thorac Surg 1999;68:2243–2247.
8 Kirklin JW: Replacement of the mitral valve for mitral incompetence. Surgery 1972;72:827–836.
9 Grewal KS, Malkowski MJ, Piracha AR, Astbury JC, Kramer CM, Dianzumba S, Reichek N: Effect of general anesthesia on the severity of mitral regurgitation by transesophageal echocardiography. Am J Cardiol 2000;85:199–203.
10 Chen FY, Adams DH, Aranki SF, Collins JJ Jr, Couper GS, Rizzo RJ, Cohn LH: Mitral valve repair in cardiomyopathy. Circulation 1998;98(suppl):11124–11127.
11 Thourani VH, Weintraub WS, Craver JM, Jones EL, Gott JP, Brown M, Puskas JD, Guyton RA: Influence of concomitant CABG and urgent/emergent status on mitral valve replacement surgery. Ann Thorac Surg 2000;70:778–784.
12 Cohn LH, Rizzo RJ, Adams DH, Couper GS, Sullivan TE, Collins JJ Jr, Aranki SF: The effect of pathophysiology on the surgical treatment of ischemic mitral regurgitation: Operative and late risks of repair versus replacement. Eur J Cardiothorac Surg 1995;9:568–674.

Lawrence H. Cohn, MD, Chief, Division of Cardiac Surgery Brigham and Women's Hospital,
75 Francis Street, Boston, MA 02115 (USA)
Tel. +1 617 7327678, Fax +1 617 7326559

Borer JS, Isom OW (eds): Pathophysiology, Evaluation and Management of Valvular Heart Diseases.
Adv Cardiol. Basel, Karger, 2002, vol 39, pp 157–163

Concomitant Mitral Repair at the Time of Coronary Artery Bypass Grafting – The 'Con' Point of View

Shawn L. Tittle, George Tolis, John A. Elefteriades

Department of Cardiothoracic Surgery, Yale University School of Medicine, New Haven, Conn., USA

The issue of whether or not to intervene for mitral valve insufficiency in a patient undergoing revascularization for ischemic cardiomyopathy is a difficult one. These patients often suffer from moderate to severe left ventricular (LV) dysfunction. Additional ischemic time for mitral repair may be poorly tolerated and may even jeopardize survival. On the other hand, without valve repair, the patient may be subject to intra-operative low cardiac output and post-operative congestive heart failure. At issue also is the late impact on quality of life or survival of mitral valve repair done at the time of coronary revascularization. This paper focuses on patients with mitral insufficiency as a consequence of ischemic disease, not those with independent, but coincident, organic mitral valve disease due to other causes (e.g. rheumatic fever, endocarditis, degenerative disease).

The question of whether or not to perform concomitant valve repair or replacement at the time of coronary revascularization cannot be answered definitively on the basis of information available in the literature. This is not surprising, as prospective comparative studies have not been done and retrospective comparisons are difficult to assess due to patient variability. Nonetheless, numerous papers have been written on the topic, either agreeing or disagreeing with concomitant mitral valve repair at the time of revascularization [1–6].

Proponents of mitral valve repair for ischemic mitral valve regurgitation at the time of revascularization often cite five main points. These include the following: that patients will not survive without mitral valve repair; that the natural history of mitral regurgitation is poor; that mitral valve repair is simple; that the patient will need mitral valve repair at a later date, and that mitral valve surgery

Table 1. Literature reports of mortality in patients with coronary artery disease and mitral insufficiency with or without repair or replacement

CABG and MV replacement	
23.7%	Czer LS, Gray RJ, De Robertis MA, et al: Mitral valve replacement: Impact of coronary artery disease and determinants of prognosis after revascularization. Circulation 1984;70:198–207
15%	He GW, Hughes CF, McCaughan B, et al: Mitral valve replacement combined with coronary artery operation: Determinants of early and late results. Ann Thorac Surg 1991;51:916–922
21%	Izhar U, Daly RC, Dearani JA, et al: Mitral valve replacement or repair after previous coronary artery bypass grafting. Circulation 1999;100:84–89
CABG and MV repair	
9.5%	Cohn LH, Rizzo RJ, Adams DH, et al: The effect of pathophysiology on the surgical treatment of ischemic mitral regurgitation: Operative and late risks of repair versus replacement. Eur J Cardiothorac Surg 1995;9:568–574
11%	Duarte IG, Murphy CO, Kosinski AS, et al: Late survival after valve operation in patients with LV dysfunction. Ann Thorac Surg 1997;64: 1089–1095
9.1%	Lawrie GM: Mitral valve replacement. Current recommendations and long-term results. Cardiol Clin 1998;16:437–448
CABG alone	
3%	Duarte IG, Shen Y, MacDonald MJ, et al: Treatment of moderate mitral regurgitation and coronary disease by coronary bypass alone: Late results. Ann Thorac Surg 1999;68:426–430
5%	Elefteriades JA, Morales DL, Gradel C, et al. Results of coronary artery bypass grafting by a single surgeon in patients with LV ejection fractions < or = 30%. Am J Cardiol 1997;79:1573–1578

is difficult to do late after coronary artery bypass grafting (CABG). We argue that survival is acceptable without mitral valve repair; that the natural history is acceptable with coronary revascularization alone; that the addition of mitral valve repair is not without considerable risk; that mitral valve repair is rarely required late, and that mitral valve repair and replacement can, in fact, be performed safely at a late date. We believe that ischemic mitral regurgitation is a disease of the left ventricle, not the mitral valve, and accordingly can be addressed by improving the left ventricle itself via revascularization.

Table 1 presents a review of selected papers on surgical therapy of patients with mitral insufficiency undergoing coronary revascularization. It can be seen that, even in recent series, the mortality risk of revascularization combined with mitral repair or replacement remains considerable (9.1–23.7%).

At the extremes of mitral valve regurgitation, the treatment plans are well supported. Mitral regurgitation of 1+ does not require valve repair, while regurgitation of 4+ does require repair. However, in the 'gray area' of 2+ or 3+ MR, problems are encountered in determining the patients for whom repair of the mitral valve is appropriate. One problem is that the exact severity of mitral regurgitation is difficult to assess. Echocardiogram often underestimates ischemic mitral regurgitation, and angiography is qualitative and imprecise [7]. Ischemic mitral regurgitation also varies, depending on the amount of ischemia the left ventricle has at any given time, and on the loading conditions. An example of this is seen in the operating room, where the ischemic mitral regurgitation is often falsely underestimated, because ischemia is minimized and preload and afterload are optimized.

Another problem with determining treatment for ischemic mitral regurgitation is that the pathologic anatomy of the disease is variable and incompletely understood. Individual cases may have papillary muscle dysfunction, shortening, lengthening, or displacement. The patient may have annular dilatation, LV remodeling, decreased LV contractile force, or superimposed intercurrent organic valvular diseases. Leaflet motion may be normal, excessive, or restricted. In the case of normal motion, a ring is thought more appropriate. In the case of excess motion, a Carpentier-type repair is warranted. In the case of restricted motion, some suggest placement of a small ring. The choice of precise surgical intervention is not trivial. The difficulty lies in prescribing a single treatment, that of mitral valve repair or replacement, for a process so variable, but originating from a single factor – LV ischemia. Also, very little attention has been placed on evaluation of the true efficacy of mitral valve repair at the time of coronary revascularization in correcting current and preventing future mitral regurgitation. The available data is not uniformly encouraging. Perrier [8] has found that with large ventricles, no technique may be effective.

Yale Experience

Certain findings in the Yale low ejection fraction (EF) CABG experience bear indirectly on the question at hand. We have carefully studied outcomes in a precisely delineated group of patients with advanced LV dysfunction undergoing CABG. Mitral insufficiency is very common in these patients.

Patients were included only if EF was ≤30%. Only angiographic or equilibrium radionuclide angiography (ERNA) EF were accepted as adequate documentation of this advanced level of LV dysfunction. Patients undergoing concomitant valve or aneurysm surgery were purposely excluded so that the impact of CABG alone could be assessed. Patients with generalized, proximal, severe coronary artery disease and adequate distal targets were accepted for surgery. No objective

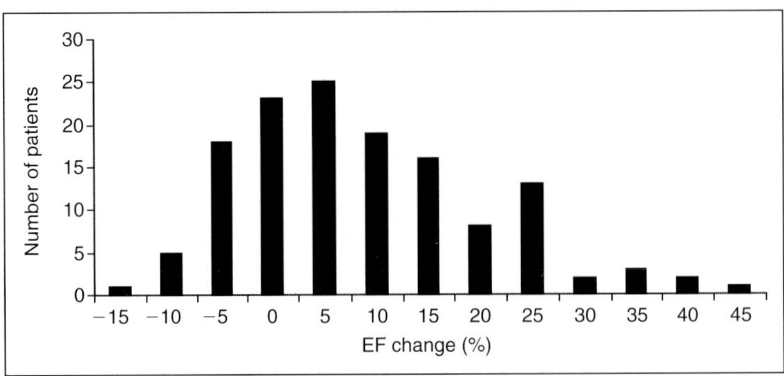

Fig. 1. Change in EF, pre- to post-operatively, in patients with CABG alone. Note that the vast majority of patients showed EF improvement, suggesting that reversible dysfunction is nearly ubiquitous [adapted from 11, with permission].

documentation of myocardial ischemia or viability was required. Sixty-six percent of patients manifested pre-operative congestive heart failure and 25% had frank pulmonary edema. Mean EF was 23% (range 10–30%).

Of these patients, 87.5% ($n = 159$) had pre-operative mitral insufficiency of 2+, or 3+ (no 4+) by angiography or echocardiography. Only 12.5% of these patients ($n = 23$) had 0–1+ mitral insufficiency.

Pertinent findings from our carefully monitored experience with this group of patients, vis-à-vis the question at hand, are the following (mean follow-up 64 months) [9–13]: (1) Operative mortality was low (5.3% in all patients, 2.3% in patients not in ICU at the time of operation). (2) CHF category improved dramatically (NYHA class 3.4–1.7) ($p < 0.05$). (3) EF improved dramatically from 23 to 34% ($p < 0.01$). EF improved in nearly all patients, even without requirement for demonstrable pre-operative ischemic zones (fig. 1). EF improvement was maintained at redetermination at 5 years. (4) Long-term survival was excellent (87, 75 and 60% at 1, 3 and 5 years respectively) compared to general expectations for this category of patients. (5) No patients required subsequent mitral valve surgery. (6) No patients went on to heart transplantation. (7) In those patients with extreme LV dilation (LVESVI $> 100\,cm/m^2$), ventricular volume actually decreased post-revascularization from 175 to $144\,cm/m^2$ ($p < 0.04$).

We believe that this low mortality rate in high-risk patients revascularized without mitral valve repair is unsurpassed by clinical series incorporating valve repair. Similarly, we are not aware of long-term survival data with repair which surpasses these data without repair. We believe the improvement realized in CHF reflects improvement in LV function as well as implying no significant clinical detriment from not approaching the mitral valve directly.

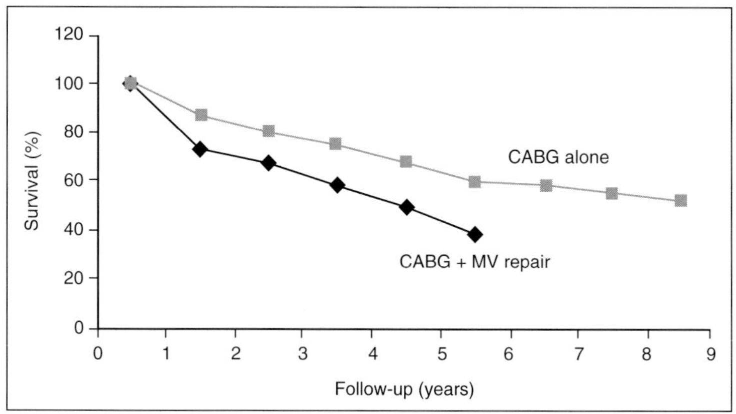

Fig. 2. Comparison of survival in patients who underwent CABG alone vs. CABG and MV repair [adapted from 5, 9, with permission].

It is known that in patients with chronic ischemic disease, mitral insufficiency is caused by regional dysfunction of LV wall segments subtending the papillary muscles as well as by LV distortion from dilation. The Yale series of CABG without mitral repair clearly improved ischemia (increased EF thought reflective of 'reanimation' of ischemic zones) and produced beneficial reverse remodeling of LV dilation. Both these factors, improvement in ischemia and return of ventricular volume toward normal, would be expected to impact beneficially on mitral regurgitation. However, this remains to be determined. We believe that the symptomatic improvement, dramatic and sustained improvement in LV function, and good long-term survival realized in this series of sole revascularization argues against the necessity for a direct surgical approach to the mitral valve in ischemic mitral insufficiency with moderate mitral regurgitation.

Of course, there was no control group of patients having concomitant mitral valve surgery in this series. Nonetheless, other literature supports this position. Guyton's group [2] demonstrated, in the largest study of this type in the literature (n = 116), that treatment of coronary artery disease and 3+ mitral regurgitation with CABG alone had an operative mortality of 3.4% and a 5-year survival of 77%. The comparison group of patients with coronary artery disease and moderate mitral regurgitation who were treated with CABG and mitral valve replacement had an operative mortality of 25% and 5-year survival of 31%. In figure 2, we plot long-term survival in our patients with moderate mitral insufficiency treated by CABG alone next to that of CABG with mitral valve repair from the data of Cohn et al. [5]. No survival benefit from repair is evident.

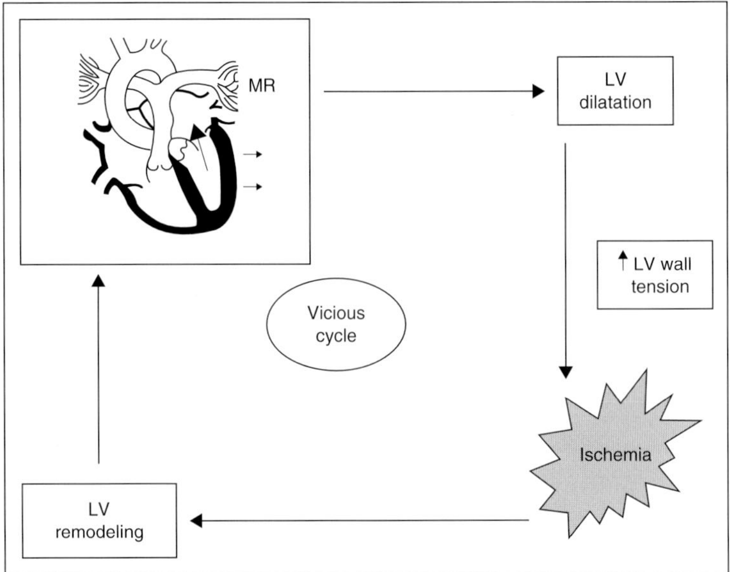

Fig. 3. Diagrammatic representation of the vicious cycle of mitral valve regurgitation leading to myocardial ischemia, which in turn leads to further mitral valve regurgitation.

A small subset of patients may have residual significant mitral valve regurgitation. Cohn's group [14] described mitral valve repair late after CABG, noting that the operation could be done with minimal complications. We have also had an excellent experience with a right thoracotomy approach for those rare instances in which mitral valve surgery needs to be performed with patent grafts from prior CABG [15]. These studies show that the patients with residual 3–4+ MR have a reliable treatment option should CABG alone fail to treat the underlying MR.

Conclusion

On the basis of our literature review and the observations from our own series of patients, we believe that patients with 2+ or 3+ MR can be operated with coronary revascularization alone with excellent short- and long-term expectations. We do not object in any way to concomitant mitral valve repair, but we believe that indications and benefits are unsubstantiated. We believe that ischemic mitral insufficiency is a disease not of the mitral valve, but rather of the left ventricle. We have evidence that revascularization alone improves the left ventricle (both function and size), and thus directly approaches the culprit component in ischemic mitral insufficiency. In terms of Perrier's diagrammatic depiction of the vicious cycle in which ischemic mitral regurgitation begets further mitral regurgitation (fig. 3), CABG alone attacks both left ventricle ischemia and left ventricle dilatation. By improving the function, size and shape of the left ventricle, CABG alone improves and controls ischemic mitral regurgitation.

References

1 Chen FY, Adams DH, Aranki SF, Collins JJ, Couper GS, Rizzo RJ, Cohn LH: Mitral valve repair in cardiomyopathy. Circulation 1998;98(suppl):124–127.

2 Duarte IG, Shen Y, MacDonald MJ, Jones EL, Craver JM, Guyton RA: Treatment of moderate mitral regurgitation and coronary artery disease by coronary artery bypass alone: Late results. Ann Thorac Surg 1999;68:426–430.

3 Christenson JT, Simonet F, Maurice J, Bloch A, Velebit V, Schmuziger M: Mitral regurgitation in patients with coronary artery disease and low left ventricular ejection fractions. How should it be treated? Texas Heart Inst J 1995;22:243–249.

4 Bolling SF: Mitral valve reconstruction in elderly ischemic patients. Chest 1996;109:35–40.

5 Cohn LH, Rizzo RJ, Adams DH, Couper GS, Sullivan TE, Collins JJ Jr, Aranki SF: The effect of pathophysiology on the surgical treatment of ischemic mitral regurgitation: Operative and late risks of repair versus replacement. Eur J Cardiothorac Surg 1995;9:568–574.

6 Duarte IG, Murphy CO, Kosinski AS, Jones EL, Craver JM, Gott JP, Guyton RA: Late survival after valve operation in patients with left ventricle dysfunction. Ann Thorac Surg 1997;64: 1089–1095.

7 Thomson HL, Enriquez-Sarano M: Echocardiographic assessment of mitral regurgitation. Cardiol Rev 2001;9:210–216.

8 Perrier P: American Association for Thoracic Surgery Meeting, 2001.

9 Elefteriades JA, Morales DL, Gradel C, Tollis G, Levi E, Zaret BL: Results of coronary artery bypass grafting by a single surgeon in patients with left ventricular ejection fractions < or = 30%. Am J Cardiol 1997;79:1573–1578.

10 Kim RW, Ugurlu BS, Tereb DA, Wackers FJ, Tellides G, Elefteriades JA: Effect of left ventricular volume on results of coronary artery bypass grafting. Am J Cardiol 2000;86:1261–1264.

11 Elefteriades JA, Tolis G, Levi EK, Mills K, Zaret BL: Coronary artery bypass surgery in severe left ventricular dysfunction: Excellent survival with improved ejection fraction and functional state. J Am Coll Cardiol 1993;22:1411–1417.

12 Tolis G, Elefteriades JA: Coronary artery bypass grafting for ischemic cardiomyopathy produces left ventricular ejection fraction improvement sustained for the long term. American Heart Association Meeting, 2001.

13 Tolis G, Korkolis D, Kopf G, Elefteriades J: Revascularization alone (without mitral valve repair) suffices in patients with advanced ischemic cardiomyopathy and mild to moderate mitral regurgitation. Society of Thoracic Surgeons Annual Meeting, 2002.

14 Byrne JG, Aranki SF, Adams DH, Rizzo RJ, Couper GS, Cohn LH: Mitral valve surgery after previous CABG with functioning IMA grafts. Ann Thorac Surg 1999;68:2243–2247.

15 Braxton JH, Higgins RSD, Schwann TA, Sanchez JA, Dewar ML, Kopf GS, Hammond GL, Elefteriades JA: Reoperative mitral valve surgery via right thoracotomy: Decreased blood loss and improved hemodynamics. J Heart Valve Dis 1996;5:169–173.

John A. Elefteriades, MD, Department of Cardiothoracic Surgery,
Yale University School of Medicine, 333 Ceder Street, 121 FMB,
New Haven, CT 06510-3206 (USA)

Borer JS, Isom OW (eds): Pathophysiology, Evaluation and Management of Valvular Heart Diseases.
Adv Cardiol. Basel, Karger, 2002, vol 39, pp 164–172

Minimally Invasive Valve Surgery: Evolution of Technique and Clinical Results

Ram Sharony, Eugene A. Grossi, Greg H. Ribakove, Patricia Ursomanno, Stephen B. Colvin, Aubery C. Galloway

Division of Cardiothoracic Surgery, Department of Surgery, New York University School of Medicine, New York, N.Y., USA

Experimental work leading to the introduction of minimally invasive valve surgery (MIVS) began in the laboratories at Stanford University [1] and New York University (NYU) [2–4] in 1994. The first clinical cases [5–7] were performed in 1995–96. During the following years, several centers started to perform mitral and aortic valve procedures through various less invasive operative approaches, utilizing mini-thoracotomy and sternotomy incisions [8–16]. MIVS has the potential of reducing overall surgical trauma, attenuating pain, lessening complications, shortening the length of hospital stay and reducing patient recovery time. An immediately obvious advantage to the technique is the ability to lessen the insult to the chest wall and improve the cosmetic result. Introduction of MIVS technique required significant modification of both cardiac surgical technique and technology and, more significantly, required the introduction of a more coordinated multidisciplinary approach [17, 18].

MIVS is performed through a small surgical access and requires connection of at least part of the cardiopulmonary bypass circuit to peripheral vessels. The original percutaneous cardiopulmonary bypass and myocardial protection system (Port Access System) was developed by industry and tested at Stanford University [19] and NYU [2–4]. The Port Access technology is an endovascular system consisting of femoral arterial cannula, a femoral venous return cannula, a retrograde cardioplegia delivery catheter and an endoaortic occlusion device (endoclamp). The current clinical set-up for minimally invasive Port Access mitral surgery is illustrated in figure 1. For MIVS, many of the catheters are placed by the anesthesiologist using intra-operative transesophageal echocardiographic guidance (fig. 2) [20].

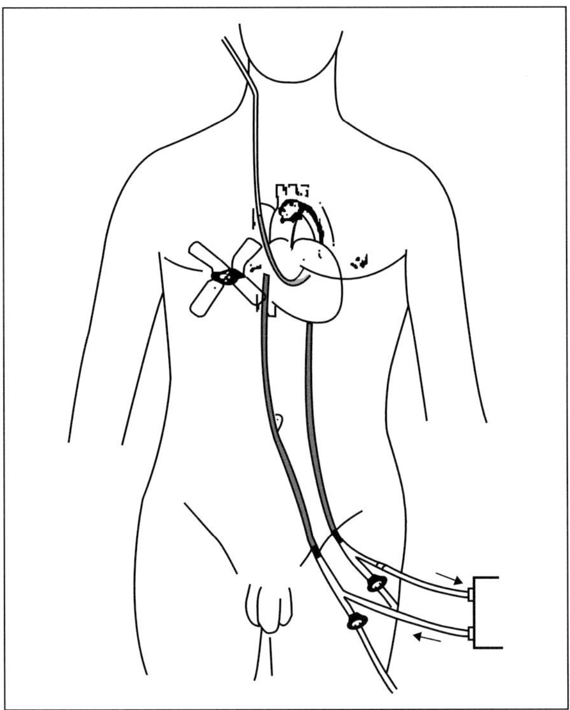

Fig. 1. Set-up for minimally invasive Port Access mitral surgery.

In the experimental laboratory it was demonstrated [2] that all measurements of regional myocardial performance were equivalent in the minimally invasive group when compared to conventional surgery and that minimally invasive Port Access bypass surgery and valve surgery were reproducible [3, 4], with complete cardiac functional recovery.

Clinical Data on Minimally Invasive Surgery

To gather scientific information and data, the multicenter Port Access International Registry (PAIR) was established. The first report by Galloway et al. [6] gave data on 1,063 patients from 121 centers, demonstrating that Port Access coronary bypass and mitral valve operations could be performed safely, with morbidity and mortality rates similar to those associated with open-chest operations. Glower et al. [21] subsequently reported data containing 1,311 isolated mitral or aortic valve surgery patients. Of these cases, 252 (19%) were aortic valve replacement (AVR), 491 (37%) were mitral valve repair (MVr), and

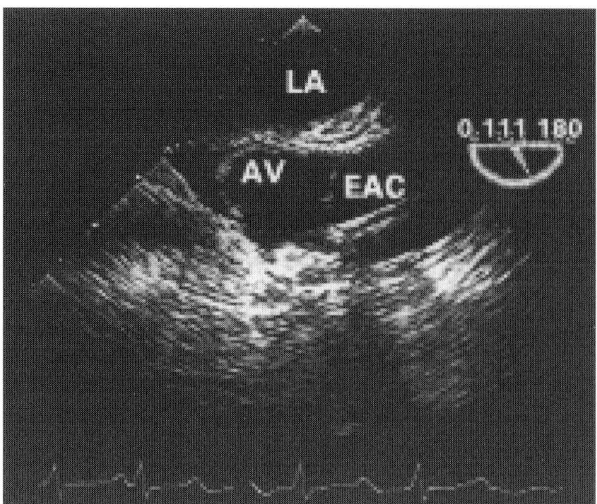

Fig. 2. Transesophageal echocardiogram (TEE) is used to position the endoaortic occlusion balloon in the ascending aorta. This longitudinal view of the ascending aorta shows the balloon of the endoaortic occlusion catheter (EAC) inflated 2–3 cm above the aortic valve (AV). The left atrium (LA) is also seen.

Table 1. NYU experience in MIVS from June 1996 up to December 2000 includes 992 patients who underwent MVP, MVR and AVR or combined procedures

Procedure	Patients, n	Mortality, %
Mitral repair	376	1.0
Mitral replacement	131	6.0
Aortic replacement	282	5.1
Multivalve/combined	203	8.8

568 (43%) were mitral valve replacement (MVR). Aortic valve procedures were performed predominantly by means of a partial sternotomy (40%) or a right anterior mini-thoracotomy (47%), and mitral valve operations were performed through a right anterior (87%) or a left lateral (10%) mini-thoracotomy. Operative mortality was 4.4% (11/252) for AVR, 1.6% (8/491) for MVr, and 5.5% (31/568) for MVR. Causes of death were generally patient-related and not a consequence of the minimally invasive approach.

The largest experience with MIVS is from NYU, with 992 patients undergoing a minimally invasive valve operation between June 1996 and December 2000 (table 1). The vast majority of patients undergoing MI-AVR were more

Table 2. Late follow-up studies performed on 376 patients undergoing MI-MVr

	n	Mortality	5-Year VR	5-Year reoperation	Cardiac survival
MIS	376	1.0%	94%	96%	97%

MIS = Minimally invasive surgery, VR = valve-related complications.

than 70 years of age, where the advantages of avoiding a sternotomy incision were thought to be especially significant. For isolated mitral valve procedures, among 407 patients undergoing MVr or MVR, the operative mortality was 2.0%, the average ventilation time was 11 h, the average ICU time was 20 h, and the average hospital stay was 5.5 days. Late follow-up studies were preformed on the 376 patients undergoing minimally invasive mitral valve repair (MI-MVr), demonstrating a 5-year cardiac survival of 97%, a 5-year freedom from reoperation of 96%, and a 5-year freedom from all valve-related complications of 94% (table 2). These results are equivalent to those previously reported after conventional valve repair [22].

In order to more precisely analyze the intermediate term echocardiographic results after MIVS [23], 100 consecutive patients undergoing MI-MVr were compared with 100 patients who had MVr with a conventional sternotomy. Both groups were similar in age and ejection fraction. There was 1.0% hospital mortality with the sternotomy approach and 0% with the minimally invasive approach. Follow-up revealed that residual mitral insufficiency was similar between the minimally invasive and sternotomy approaches; the 1-year echocardiographic score was 0.79 and 0.77 respectively (0 to 3 scale). Likewise, the cumulative freedom from reoperation was not significantly different and the late New York Heart Association (NYHA) functional classes were equivalent between the two groups (table 3). These findings demonstrate that MI-MVr is comparable to conventional surgery in terms of survival, repair durability and freedom from valve-related complication (fig. 3).

Patient Benefits

Several studies from NYU have evaluated potential differences in complication rates, pain and recovery time after minimally invasive versus conventional cardiac surgery. Grossi et al. [24] reported results in a case-control study

Table 3. Minimally invasive valve repair is comparable to standard sternotomy

	SS (n = 100)	MIS (n = 100)
Age, years	55	57
Hospital mortality, %	1	0
Residual MR (1 year)	0.79	0.77
NYHA (1 year)	1.6	1.3
Freedom reoperation, %	93	95

SS = Standard sternotomy, MIS = minimally invasive surgery, MR = mitral regurgitation.

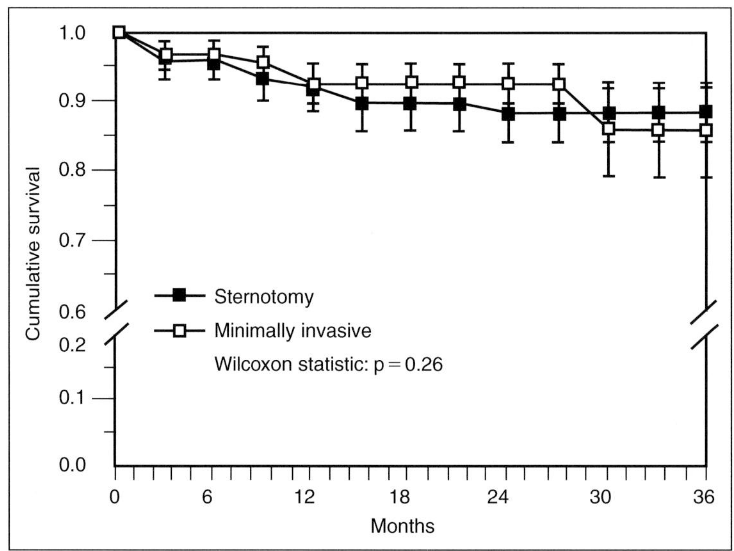

Fig. 3. Cumulative survival from all valve-related complications (anticoagulant, endocarditis, and thromoembolic) and mitral valve reoperations.

of 109 patients undergoing isolated aortic or mitral valve surgery using the Port Access minimally invasive technique, compared with 88 patients having conventional valve surgery. Age, NYHA functional classes, valve type, surgeon, previous cardiac surgery, and the presence of congestive heart failure were matched in the two groups. Hospital mortality was not significantly different, but the minimally invasive patients had a shorter hospital stay (7 vs. 9 days; p = 0.001), a decreased number of combined septic, wound and pulmonary

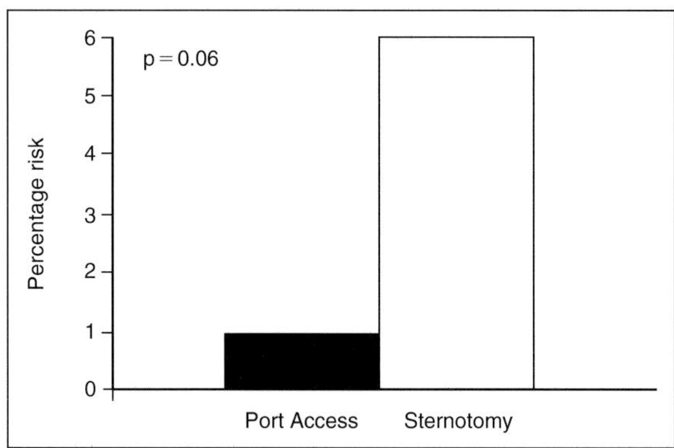

Fig. 4. Incidence of sepsis or wound complication in MIVS.

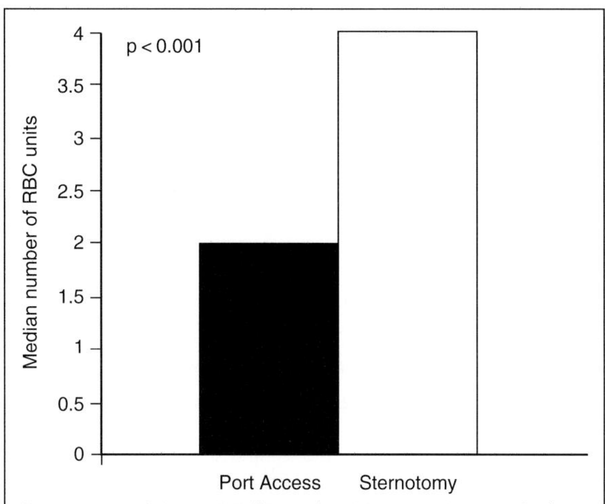

Fig. 5. Blood cell transfusion (including autologous) in MIVS.

complications (0.9% for minimally invasive vs. 5.7% for sternotomy; $p = 0.05$; fig. 4) and significantly fewer blood transfusions ($p = 0.02$; fig. 5). Similar benefits were separately demonstrated in the geriatric population [25], where the differences seem to be even more profound. Thus, clinical studies have clearly demonstrated significant benefits for patients undergoing minimally invasive surgery. The most significant benefits are less need for blood, less pain, fewer septic wound and pulmonary complications, and a shorter hospital stay.

Likewise, post-operative pain, stress response, rapidity of recovery, and quality of life were compared in a study evaluating Port Access minimally invasive

CABG versus conventional CABG [26]. Repeated measures analysis of variance showed lower pain scale ratings over the first 4 post-operative weeks in the minimally invasive group ($p < 0.001$), less muscle soreness, shortness of breath, fatigue and loss of appetite at 1, 2, 4 and 8 weeks ($p < 0.05$), better pulmonary function at 1 and 3 days ($p < 0.03$) and lower norepinephrine (catecholamine stress response) levels at days 1, 2 and 3 ($p = 0.005$). The Duke Activity Scale questionnaire to evaluate functional recovery validated that minimally invasive patients were better able to walk 1–2 blocks at 1 week, climb stairs at 1 and 2 weeks, perform light or moderate housework at 1 and 2 weeks, and engage in moderate recreational activities and perform heavy housework at 4 and 8 weeks ($p < 0.05$). This study demonstrated that minimally invasive cardiac surgery through a mini-thoracotomy resulted in less pain, better post-operative lung function, attenuation of stress response, improved early post-operative functional status, and a shorter recovery time when compared with patients requiring a sternotomy incision.

Conclusions

In summary, MIVS treatment of valvular heart disease has expanded exponentially over the last several years. The minimally invasive approach can be used routinely for both AVR and MVr or MVR, as well as for many patients with multivalve pathology. Clinical studies series have demonstrated that MIVS has a low morbidity and mortality and achieves equivalent functional and echocardiographic outcomes to those obtained with conventional surgery. Measurable patient benefits include less pain, fewer blood transfusions, fewer septic wound and pulmonary complications, a shorter recovery time, improved functional recovery and a better cosmetic result. MIVS is readily reproducible and the technique should be considered the preferential treatment for many patients requiring valvular heart surgery.

References

1 Pompili MF, Stevens JH, Burdon TA, et al: Port Access mitral valve replacement in dogs. J Thorac Cardiovasc Surg 1996;112:1268–1274.

2 Schwartz DS, Ribakove GH, Grossi EA, Buttenheim PM, Schwartz JD, Applebaum RM, Kronzon I, Baumann FG, Colvin SB, Galloway AC: Minimally invasive mitral valve replacement: Port Access technique, feasibility and myocardial functional preservation. J Thorac Cardiovasc Surg 1997;113:1022–1030.

3 Schwartz DS, Ribakove GH, Grossi EA, Schwartz JD, Buttenheim PM, Baumann FG, Colvin SB, Galloway AC: Single and multivessel Port Access coronary artery bypass grafting with cardioplegic arrest: Technique and reproducibility. J Thorac Cardiovasc Surg 1997;114:46–52.

4 Schwartz DS, Ribakove GH, Grossi EA, Stevens JH, Siegel LC, St Goar FG, Peters WS, McLoughlin D, Baumann FG, Colvin SB, Galloway AC: Minimally invasive cardiopulmonary

bypass with cardioplegic arrest: A closed chest technique with equivalent myocardial protection. J Thorac Cardiovasc Surg 1996;111:556–566.
5 Pompili MF, Yakub A, Siegel LC, Stevens JH, Awang Y, Burdon TA: Port Access mitral valve replacement: Initial clinical experience. Circulation 1996;94(suppl 1):533.
6 Galloway AC, Ribakove GH, Grossi EA, Applebaum RM, Colvin SB: Minimally invasive Port Access valvular surgery: Initial clinical experience. Circulation 1997(suppl 1):508.
7 Colvin SB, Galloway AC, Ribakove G, Grossi EA, Zakow P, Buttenheim PM, Baumann FG: Port Access mitral valve surgery: Summary of results. J Card Surg 1998;13:286–289.
8 Byrne JG, Hsin MK, Adams DH, Aklog L, Aranki SF, Couper GS, Rizzo RJ, Cohn LH: Minimally invasive direct access heart valve surgery. J Card Surg 2000;15:21–34.
9 Cosgrove DM 3rd, Sabik JF, Navia JL: Minimally invasive valve operations. Ann Thorac Surg 1998;65:1535–1538.
10 Gundry SR, Shattuck OH, Razzouk AJ, del Rio MJ, Sardari FF, Bailey LL: Facile minimally invasive cardiac surgery via ministernotomy. Ann Thorac Surg 1998;65:1100–1104.
11 Schroeyers P, Wellens F, De Geest R, Degrieck I, Van Praet F, Vermeulen Y, Vanermen H: Minimally invasive video-assisted mitral valve surgery: Our lessons after a 4-year experience. Ann Thorac Surg 2001;72:S1050–S1054.
12 Szwerc MF, Benckart DH, Wiechmann RJ, Savage EB, Szydlowski GW, Magovern GJ Jr, Magovern JA: Partial versus full sternotomy for aortic valve replacement. Ann Thorac Surg 1999; 68:2209–2213.
13 Glower DD, Landolfo KP, Clements F, Debruijn NP, Stafford-Smith M, Smith PK, Duhaylongsod F: Mitral valve operation via Port Access versus median sternotomy. Eur J Cardiothorac Surg 1998;14(suppl 1):S143–S147.
14 Felger JE, Chitwood WR Jr, Nifong LW, Holbert D: Evolution of mitral valve surgery: Toward a totally endoscopic approach. Ann Thorac Surg 2001;72:1203–1208.
15 Mohr FW, Falk V, Diegeler A, Walther T, van Son JA, Autschbach R: Minimally invasive Port Access mitral valve surgery. J Thorac Cardiovasc Surg 1998;115:567–574.
16 Gulielmos V, Wagner FM, Waetzig B, Solowjowa N, Tugtekin SM, Schroeder C, Schueler S: Clinical experience with minimally invasive coronary artery and mitral valve surgery with the advantage of cardiopulmonary bypass and cardioplegic arrest using the Port Access technique. World J Surg 1999;23:480–485.
17 Applebaum RM, Cutler WM, Bhardwaj N, Colvin SB, Galloway AC, Ribakove GH, Grossi EA, Schwartz DS, Anderson RV, Tunick PA, Kronzon I: Utility of transesophageal echocardiography during Port Access minimally invasive cardiac surgery. Am J Cardiol 1998;82:183–188.
18 Kort S, Applebaum RM, Grossi EA, Baumann FG, Colvin SB, Galloway AC, Ribakove GH, Steinberg BM, Piedad B, Tunick PA, Kronzon I: Minimally invasive aortic valve replacement: Echocardiographic and clinical results. Am Heart J 2001;142:476–481.
19 Stevens JH, Burdon TA, Peters WS, Siegel LC, Pompili MF, Vierra MA, St Goar FG, Ribakove GH, Mitchell RS, Reitz BA: Port Access coronary artery bypass grafting: A proposed surgical method. J Thorac Cardiovasc Surg 1996;111:567–573.
20 Applebaum RM, Colvin SB, Galloway AC, Ribakove GH, Grossi EA, Tunick PA, Kronzon I: The role of transesophageal echocardiography during Port Access minimally invasive cardiac surgery: A new challenge for the echocardiographer. Echocardiography 1999;16:595–602.
21 Glower DD, Siegel LC, Frischmeyer KJ, Galloway AC, Ribakove GH, Grossi EA, Robinson NB, Ryan WH, Colvin SB: Predictors of outcome in a multicenter Port Access valve registry. Ann Thorac Surg 2000;70:1054–1059.
22 Spencer FC, Galloway AC, Grossi EA, et al: Recent developments and evolving techniques of mitral valve reconstruction. Ann Thorac Surg 1998;65:307–313.
23 Grossi EA, LaPietra A, Ribakove GH, Delianides J, Esposito R, Culliford AT, Derivaux CC, Applebaum RM, Kronzon I, Steinberg BM, Baumann FG, Galloway AC, Colvin SB: Minimally invasive versus sternotomy approaches for mitral reconstruction: Comparison of intermediate term results. J Thorac Cardiovasc Surg 2001;121:708–713.
24 Grossi EA, Galloway AC, Ribakove GH, Zakow PK, Derivaux CC, Baumann FG, Schwesinger D, Colvin SB: Impact of minimally invasive valvular heart surgery: A case-control study. Ann Thorac Surg 2001;71:807–810.

25 Grossi EA, Galloway AC, Ribakove GH, Buttenheim PM, Esposito R, Baumann FG, Colvin SB: Minimally invasive Port Access surgery reduces operative morbidity for valve replacement in the elderly. Heart Surg Forum 1999;2:212–215.
26 Grossi EA, Zakow PK, Ribakove G, Kallenbach K, Ursomanno P, Gradek CE, Baumann FG, Colvin SB, Galloway AC: Comparison of post-operative pain, stress response and quality of life in Port Access vs. standard sternotomy coronary bypass patients. Eur J Cardiothorac Surg 1999;16(suppl 2):S39–S42.

Aubrey C. Galloway, MD, New York University Medical Center, Skirball Institute,
Suite 9V HCC-6D, 550 First Avenue, New York, NY 10016 (USA)

Borer JS, Isom OW (eds): Pathophysiology, Evaluation and Management of Valvular Heart Diseases.
Adv Cardiol. Basel, Karger, 2002, vol 39, pp 173–183

Blood Conservation: Is It Working?

Karl H. Krieger

Department of Cardiothoracic Surgery and The Howard Gilman Institute of Valvular Heart Diseases, Weill Medical College of Cornell University, New York-Presbyterian Hospital-New York Weill Cornell Medical Center, New York, N.Y., USA

Historically, blood transfusion has always been associated with cardiac surgery. In the late 1960s and early 1970s, patients undergoing cardiovascular surgery were routinely typed and cross-matched with 10 units of blood. Before discharge, most of the blood was utilized. During the early 1980s, 8 units of red blood cells (RBC) were routinely prepared and cardiac surgeons and cardiologists alike had a low threshold for transfusing blood in the postoperative setting. In 1985 this laissez-faire attitude changed. We were startled by information regarding blood transfusions, the HIV virus and AIDS; suddenly we became aware of this new danger associated with blood transfusion practices. As part of a state-wide transfusion 'look back' program in New York, surgeons received a list of patients in whom transfusion with HIV-tainted blood was suspected. Many of the listed patients had passed away at the time we contacted their families. Death certificates stated that they had died of hepatitis, pneumonia or multisystem failure. As a result, enormous pressure was placed on cardiac programs and cardiac surgeons to restrict the use of blood. Some patients refused coronary artery bypass surgery without a guarantee that they would not need transfusion. Simultaneously, facing the need for cost reductions, hospital and blood bank administrators totaled the cost of blood components used in their cardiac surgery program and asked that transfusion practices be re-examined. In addition, religious groups that refuse blood transfusion, such as Jehovah Witnesses, wanted cardiac surgery to become more available to their members. Because of these factors, most cardiac centers instituted 'blood conservation' programs.

At The New York Hospital, we initiated a retrospective study to establish a baseline to evaluate our blood usage patterns. We reviewed 100 consecutive coronary artery bypass patients, and found that the average coronary artery bypass

Table 1. Transfusion risks 1992

Major	Minor
HIV disease (1 : 100,000–1 : 125,000)	Febrile reaction
Hepatitis B (1 : 200,000)	Graft vs. host disease (1 : 1 million)
Hepatitis C (1 : 2,000–1 : 6,000)	Delayed hemolytic transfusion reaction (1 : 33,000)
Acute hemolytic transfusion reaction (1 : 33,000)	Alloimmunization
Allergic reaction (1 : 20,000)	Immunosuppression

Table 2. Transfusion costs 1992

Product	Cost
RBC (packed)	USD 220.00
Platelets (6 units)	USD 400.00
Single donor PLT (6 units)	USD 620.00
Cryoprecipitate (10 units)	USD 600.00
FFP (2 units)	USD 140.00

patient was exposed to 2.3 units of RBC and 2.9 units of fresh frozen plasma (FFP), platelets, or cryoprecipitate, for a total of 5.2 blood exposures.

Reviewing studies from other centers we found that bypass patients received as many as 13 blood exposures per patient with most exposure coming from clotting factors, not RBC [1]. Concluding that our studies were consistent with the experiences at other medical centers, we decided that we could significantly reduce exposure by designing a multimodality blood conservation program to minimize dependence on blood and blood factor transfusions.

Further review of our own data revealed that three groups of patients are at relatively high risk of homologous transfusion. These are patients of advanced age, patients with advanced and complex disease, and patients requiring reoperation. Transfusion risks fell into two categories, major and minor: *Major risks* (see table 1 for 1992 incidence rates; transfusion risk of HIV in 2001 is 1 : 500,000) include contracting HIV, hepatitis B, hepatitis C, acute hemolytic reaction, and allergic reaction. *Minor risks* included febrile reaction, graft-versus-host disease, delayed hemolytic transfusion reaction, alloimmunization and immunosuppression.

Transfusion costs to third-party payers and patients were considerable. In New York City the average cost of a unit of packed RBC was USD 220, 6 units of platelets cost USD 400, 6 units of single donor platelets cost USD 620, 10 units of cryoprecipitate cost USD 600 and 2 units of FFP cost USD 140 (table 2).

Table 3. Transfusion costs 1992

400,000 open-heart procedures per year
Red cells (2.3 units/patient): 2.3 units × USD 220/unit × 400,000 = USD 202,000,000
Platelets, FFP, cryoprecipitate (2.9 units/patient): 2.9 units × USD 75/unit × 400,000 = USD 87,000,000
Total transfusion cost per year USD ~ 300,000,000

Table 4. Preoperative blood conservation

Maximize available red blood cell mass
- Preoperative autologous donation
- Iron supplementation
- Erythropoietin
- Minimize laboratory testing and other procedural blood losses

Optimize coagulation status

Approximately 400,000 open-heart procedures are done yearly in the USA. If one employs the cost data, above, and assumes, as previously noted, that the average patient is transfused with 2.3 units of RBC and 2.9 units of platelets, cryoprecipitate, and FFP (average cost for these products = USD 75 per unit), then the total transfusion cost for all payers combined totals approximately USD 300,000,000 yearly (table 3). The true total is probably underestimated because the total cost is based on data derived from routine coronary artery bypass patients. Patients with valvular heart disease and mixed coronary and valvular disease often have increased transfusion requirements.

To build a comprehensive, multimodality blood conservation program, we separated the patients' medical experiences into three time frames: the preoperative period, intraoperative time, and the postoperative period. Preoperative efforts (table 4) are directed towards maximizing available RBC mass. This can be done with preoperative autologous donation, a technique that has worked well in the orthopedic and general surgical population. This technique has not been widely adopted in cardiac surgical patients because the waiting period required between donation and surgery may be medically inadvisable and because the resulting anemia is unsafe in certain cardiac patient populations. A more effective technique of increasing RBC mass involves the usage of erythropoietin and iron supplementation. Used in combination, the intravenous and subcutaneous injection of erythropoietin with iron supplementation has been very effective in increasing preoperative hemoglobin levels and total RBC mass

Table 5. Intraoperative blood conservation

Intraoperative autologous donation (IAD)
Minimize unnecessary hemodilution
Small volume cardiopulmonary bypass (CPB) circuit
Eliminate unnecessary fluid administration
Reverse autologous circuit priming (RAP)
Lowest safe transfusion trigger (15%)
Intraoperative blood salvage (cell saver)
Antifibrinolytic therapy (aprotinin, Amicar)
Meticulous surgical technique

within 5–7 days of therapy. This is a very effective technique in the Jehovah Witness patient population but is limited in the general cardiac surgical population because of its substantial cost. Therapy will often cost between USD 800 and 1,200 per patient depending on the dosage. Other preoperative techniques include minimizing laboratory testing and other procedural blood losses. Optimizing coagulation status prior to surgery is critical to prevent intraoperative and postoperative blood loss. We require a prothrombin time <13 (generally associated with INR <1.2) before proceeding with elective surgery. Stopping aspirin 10 days prior to surgery is ideal but most bypass patients have had aspirin just before surgery without negative consequences.

Intraoperative techniques have the greatest impact on our total blood conservation program (table 5). Intraoperative autologous donation (IAD) has proven to be one of the most effective techniques of blood conservation. Unlike preoperative autologous technique, removing the patient's blood in the operating room prior to cardiopulmonary bypass has been proven to be completely safe. The cardiac patient is asleep and is fully monitored with arterial and pulmonary artery lines while 10–20% of the patient's blood volume is slowly withdrawn by the anesthesia team. This blood is citrated and placed aside for retransfusion after protamine administration at the conclusion of the pump run. The patient is then transfused with 2–3 units of autologous blood, which includes 2–3 units of clotting factor and platelets. The RBC have not been traumatized by the bypass circuit and circulating blood proteins (clotting factors) have not been depleted by the oxygenator and the circuit lines. This technique was first reported by Dodrill et al. [2] in 1957 but has not been widely utilized until recently. Multiple studies have documented that its use results in decreased postoperative bleeding and in decreased transfusion requirements [3–5].

An important part of all blood conservation programs is the minimization of unnecessary hemodilution. Hemodilution often occurs during the induction of anesthesia. The transient drop in blood pressure seen during the initial stages of anesthesia is treated with volume administration. Further hemodilution occurs with initiation of cardiopulmonary bypass. Most bypass circuits contain 1,500–2,000 ml of salt-based solution (0.9% saline or lactated Ringer's), which immediately dilutes the patient's RBC mass. Hematocrits drop into the low 20s or high teens and many perfusionists routinely transfuse after initiation of bypass.

Hypotension associated with anesthesia induction can be treated with carefully administered alpha constrictor medications and protein solutions, decreasing the need for volume loading. Low volume bypass circuits (900 ml) with low volume oxygenators have been developed that significantly reduce the hemodilution seen with bypass.

A new technique called reverse autologous circuit priming (or RAPing) [6] has also been effective in minimizing the dilution effect. This technique utilizes the patient's own blood volume to prime the circuit. On some cases as little as 500 ml of prime saline are in the cardiopulmonary circuit at the time bypass is initiated. Hematocrits in these patients may be maintained in the high 20s throughout a pump run, eliminating the need for transfusion.

Re-evaluating transfusion triggers in the operating room has played an important role in our blood conservation program. Many cardiac centers routinely transfuse patients while on pump when the hematocrit falls below 20%. Packed RBC are given, keeping the hematocrit between 20 and 25%, although there is little factual data in the literature supporting the need for transfusion. A question commonly asked in many cardiac programs is 'What is the lowest safe hematocrit while on bypass?' There is no clear answer to this question. We retrospectively reviewed 3,800 bypass cases completed at New York Hospital between 1990 and 1993 examining 'lowest hematocrit on bypass' as a surgical risk factor. End points included myocardial infarction (MI), death, cerebrovascular accident (CVA), and renal failure. This study found that a perfusion hematocrit of 15% was safe for most patients when hypothermia techniques were part of the perfusion run. Patients with a history of peripheral vascular disease or patients ≥75 years old needed a perfusion HCT of ≥17%. We found that by lowering our perfusion triggers to 15 (17 in selected cases) we could eliminate the need for most transfusions on bypass. This technique is safe and is still practiced today [7].

Intraoperative blood salvage is not a new concept but is an effective technique in reducing transfusion requirements. A conscientious effort to return all lost blood to the cell saver is helpful, including blood squeezed out of lap pads. This fluid, which in years past was routinely discarded, is filtered, washed, hemoconcentrated, and then returned to the patient. Blood left in the oxygenator and perfusion lines at the end of the case are also hemoconcentrated and reinfused.

Antifibrinolytic therapy with Amicar, tranexamic acid (TA), and aprotinin routinely is practiced at our institution. Amicar and TA are both synthetic antifibrinolytics with similar pharmacologic properties, forming a reversible complex

Table 6. Postoperative blood conservation

Reinfusion of shed blood
Maximize RBC mass regeneration
Iron, nutrition
Erythropoietin
Correction of coagulopathy
Delineate 'medical' vs. 'surgical' bleeding
Antifibrinolytics, DDAVP
Transfusion guidelines
Minimize unnecessary blood loss

with either plasminogen or plasmin. These drugs block the premature dissolution of the normal fibrin clot. Aprotinin is a serine-protease inhibitor and intervenes in the coagulation cascade at multiple loci resulting in antiplasmin and antikallikrein effects during cardiopulmonary bypass. Multiple studies demonstrate a decrease in blood loss after cardiopulmonary bypass with the routine use of these drugs [8, 9].

Meticulous surgical techniques with a careful non-hurried post-pump search for bleeding sites is a cornerstone of all blood conservation programs. Surgical bleeding should be eliminated before the chest is closed because it will not stop with only a pharmacological approach.

Postoperative therapeutic approaches have a major role in a blood conservation program (table 6). Reinfusion of shed mediastinal blood has been practiced at many cardiac centers since the 1980s. This technique is safe and helps preserve RBC volume. RBC regeneration can be stimulated with postoperative erythropoietin. This technique, combined with iron and folate administration, can be very effective in correcting postoperative anemia. Erythropoietin given preoperatively will stimulate an early rise in postoperative hemoglobin levels. Correction of postoperative coagulopathy is a critical step in preventing postoperative blood loss. Heparin neutralization with protamine should be monitored with frequent activated clotting times (ACT). Antifibrinolytic agents like Amicar, TA and aprotinin should be continued. Desmopressin acetate (DDAVP), a synthetic analogue of the hormone vasopressin, has been widely studied in postoperative patients and may be beneficial in treating patient subsets at increased risk of bleeding.

Having specific transfusion guidelines again plays an important role in reducing blood overutilization. It is customary in many cardiac centers to immediately transfuse patients with substantial bleeding during the first hour after operation. Shotgun therapy with packed RBC, FFP and platelets is commonly utilized. We found that instituting specific guidelines for blood and factor therapy

Table 7. Treatment algorithm for excessive bleeding during the intraoperative post-CPB and postoperative periods

Quantity of bleeding

Intraoperative post-CPB period

Severe 'microvascular' bleeding with suspected (based on characteristics of CPB run and/or procedure performed) or documented quantitative platelet or coagulation factor deficiency

Postoperative period

Immediate bleeding

Drainage >300 ml during first hour (order products, but do not give unless #2 occurs)

Drainage >250 ml second hour (actually give ordered products)

If drainage <250 ml/h during second hour, patient is not transfused but continues to be assessed for delayed postoperative bleeding

Delayed bleeding

Drainage >200 ml during any 2 consecutive hours after the first 2 postoperative hours (platelets and/or factors ordered after the first >200 ml hour)

Drainage >100 ml over any 4 h after the first 2 postoperative hours (platelets and/or factors ordered after the third of these hours)

Treatment

Rapid application of nontransfusion therapy

Transfusion therapy

Transfusion of 6 units platelets:

Platelet count <100,000

Platelet count >100,000, with nl PT (<15.0 s – i.e., for presumed severe platelet dysfunction)

Transfusion 2 units FFP:

PT >15.0 s

PTT >1.5 × control, ACT wnl or no correction with 100 mg extra protamine dose

Transfuse 10 units cryoprecipitate if 12 units platelets + 4 units FFP and still coagulopathic bleeding (PT/PTT >1.5 × nl, fibrinogen <100)

greatly reduced our blood and blood product utilization (table 7). These guidelines mandate no transfusion in the first postoperative hour unless massive blood loss is encountered. Then very specific indicators are utilized for factor transfusion. Hematocrits are maintained >22% in the early postoperative setting with a slightly higher hematocrit of 25% in the elderly (>75 years) or in patients with known peripheral vascular disease. Early return to the operating room is necessary when bleeding is massive or when total blood loss reaches 1,000 ml. Delaying longer in our experience has resulted in increased transfusion requirements and usually does not eliminate the need for re-exploration.

To evaluate the efficacy of our blood conservation program, we prospectively applied our multimodality program to 100 consecutive patients undergoing primary coronary artery bypass grafting. To assess the effects of this algorithm on bleeding, transfusion reduction and safety, we compared the results with those achieved in a similar group of patients to whom an identical set of transfusion guidelines was applied but in whom a more limited set of blood conservation measures was used. We also attempted to assess cost efficiency by comparing our patients with Diagnosis-Related Group (DRG) matched controls from our institution. This study produced impressive results [10]. Our 100 consecutive bypass patients underwent coronary artery bypass grafting without any allogenic transfusion. The control population was transfused with a mean of 2.2 units of blood per patient with 38% receiving transfusion. Postoperative blood loss at 12 h in the control group was double that in the patient test group. The total hospitalization cost for the test group in each of the three major DRG categories was equivalent to or significantly less than those in the matched controls. We concluded that a comprehensive multimodality blood conservation program (fig. 1) could significantly decrease postoperative bleeding and the need for allogenic transfusions in a safe and cost-effective manner.

Many of the guidelines established in our blood conservation program have proven difficult to maintain over a long period of time. Each physician has had his own set of clinical experiences and has specific ideas about appropriate transfusion triggers, indications for blood products, and the timing of re-exploration. New techniques like RAPing and Intraoperative Autologous Blood Donation do not appeal to all anesthesiologists and cardiac surgeons. House officers in university programs want to 'do a good job' and may be overly aggressive about treating early blood loss in the postoperative setting. Decisions in the postoperative period are made by intensivists, cardiologists, house officers, nurse practitioners and physician assistants. Cardiac surgeons often lose immediate control of their patients' management. In this setting, overtransfusion and inappropriate transfusion is commonplace.

We therefore reviewed our blood conservation program again in the year 2000 to compare our current performance with that achieved in 1992, when we first examined our blood transfusion practices. At that time we noted that the average coronary artery bypass patient was exposed to 5.2 units per patient. Patients averaged 2.3 units of transfused RBC and 2.9 units of FFP, platelets, or cryoprecipitate. During the year 2000, a total of 1,503 total pump cases were

Fig. 1. The New York Hospital-Cornell Medical College Multimodality Blood Conservation Program. Techniques and pharmacologic agents are listed under the perioperative period in which they are applied. Newer modalities which have not yet been clearly demonstrated to be of benefit or are investigational are listed in italics. LMWH = Low-molecular-weight heparin; PAF = platelet activation factor; BP = blood pressure; ACT = activated clotting time; EACA = ϵ-aminocaproic acid; DDAVP = *D*-arginine amino vasopressin; PEEP = positive end-expiratory pressure; TPA = tissue plasminogen activator.

Blood conservation summary

Preoperative

All patients:

Iron, vitamin C, Colace

Folate, vitamin B_{12}

Minimize unnecessary blood loss:
1. Pediatric blood tubes
2. Minimum lab testing algorithm
3. Return A-line flushes
4. Hemostatic technique for procedures (lines, etc.)

Selected patients:

Erythropoietin:
1. Jehovah's Witness, etc.
2. Rare blood type
3. Renal failure/insufficiency

Preoperative autologous donation (PAD):
1. 2 wk min. preoperative period
2. Epo-assisted PAD

Cessation/avoidance of medications predisposing to bleeding:
1. Aspirin
2. Heparin
3. Coumadin
4. Thrombolytic agents (TPA, etc.)

Vitamin K:
1. Hepatic disease
2. Coumadin overdose (with care)

Intraoperative

All patients:

Minimize unnecessary crystalloid/colloid use

Large volume intraop. autologous donation (IAD)

Small volume CPB circuit

Non-heme CPB circuit prime

Retrograde autologous blood prime (RAP)

Optimal anticoagulation during CPB:
1. Heparin
2. Protamine

Complete intraoperative salvage:
1. Cell saver

Optimal surgical technique/hemostasis

Minimum safe red cell transfusion trigger:
1. No ischemia risk – 15%
2. Ischemia risk – 17%

Rapid sustained warming

Residual CPB circuit blood reinfusion

Minimum safe platelet and coag. factor transfusion guidelines

Selected patients:

Aprotinin prophylaxis:
1. Reoperative procedure
2. Severe increased bleeding risk
3. Jehovah's Witness

EACA prophylaxis:
1. Moderate increased bleeding risk
2. Allergy to aprotinin

Hemofiltration:
1. Hypervolemia with low hematocrit
2. Large volume clean blood processing

Heparin bonded circuitry

Leukocyte filtration

Alternative anticoag. for CPB when heparin contraindication:
1. Hirudin
2. Ancrod
3. LMWH

Postoperative

All patients:

Shed mediastinal blood reinfusion (intermittent)

Minimum safe red cell transfusion trigger:
1. Asymptomatic – 21%
2. Symptomatic – up to 30% (1 unit at a time)

Minimum safe platelet and coag. factor transfusion guidelines

Avoidance of medications that can effect hemostasis or platelet number/function:
1. Hetastarch
2. H-2 blockers (platelet count)
3. Heparin

Minimize unnecessary blood loss:
1. Pediatric blood tubes
2. Minimum lab testing algorithm
3. Return A-line flushes
4. Hemostatic technique for procedures (lines etc.)

Selected patients:

Erythropoietin:
1. Jehovah's Witness, etc.
2. Rare blood type
3. Renal failure/insufficiency

Comprehensive postoperative bleeding protocol (based on rate of chest tube output):
1. Rapid rewarming to 38°C
2. Aggressive BP control
3. PEEP increase (10 mm Hg)
4. Elevation of head of bed
5. Delayed SMB blood reinfus
6. Diagnostic testing
   - a)STAT Labs
     1. CBC platelet count
     2. PT/PTT
     3. ACT
     4. On-site testing
   - b) Serial chest radiographs
   - c) Hemodynam. monitoring
     1. Tamponade
     2. Hypertension
     3. Hypotension
7. Pharmacologic agents
   - a) Adequate heparin reversal
   - b) EACA
   - c) DDAVP
   - d) Postoperative aprotinin
8. Minimum safe platelet and coagulation factor transfusion guidelines

Early return to the operating room for critical bleeding

Table 8. Weill Medical College of Cornell University New York Hospital Year 2000 pump cases

Cases (total 1,503)	Cases, n	Average units of RBC
Coronary artery bypass Grafting (CAB)	738	0.46
CAB + valve	168	0.89
Valve or multivalve	253	0.34

completed at the New York-Presbyterian Hospital-Weill Medical College of Cornell University; 738 coronary artery bypass patients received an average of 0.46 units of RBC, a significant decrease from average in 1992 (2.3 units), 168 coronary artery bypass plus valve patients averaged 0.89 units of RBC, and 253 valve or multivalve patients averaged 0.34 units of packed RBC (table 8).

It appears reasonable to conclude that blood conservation techniques are still practiced at the New York-Presbyterian Hospital, and there has been a significant decrease in blood utilization compared to 1992. These techniques are safe and cost-effective and it is likely that similar results can be obtained at other cardiac surgery centers. Today's medical practitioners are working at a time when politicians, patient advocate groups and managed care programs are scrutinizing the medical establishment for cost-effectiveness and quality guidelines. It behooves all physicians to provide the best possible care at the lowest possible cost. Blood conservation in cardiac surgery takes an important step toward achieving this goal.

References

1 Krieger KH, Isom OW: Blood Conservation in Cardiac Surgery. Berlin, Springer, 1998, pp 633–637.

2 Dodrill FD, Marshall N, Nyboer J, et al: The use of the heart-lung apparatus in human cardiac surgery. J Thorac Surg 1957;33:60–73.

3 Wagstaffe JG, Clarke AD, Jackson PW: Reduction of blood loss by restoration of platelet levels using fresh autologous blood after cardiopulmonary bypass. Thorax 1972;27:410–414.

4 Ochsner JL, Mills NL, Leonard GL, et al: Fresh autologous blood transfusions with extracorporeal circulation. Ann Surg 1973;177:811–817.

5 Cohn LH, Fosberg AM, Anderson WP, et al: The effects of phlebotomy, hemodilution and autologous transfusion on systemic oxygenation and whole blood utilization in open-heart surgery. Chest 1975;68:283–287.

6 Schill DM: The optimal preservation of the patient's hematocrit when CPB is required. J Extracorp Tech 1990;22:73–78.

7 Krieger KH, Isom OW: Blood Conservation in Cardiac Surgery. Berlin, Springer, 1998, pp 397–438.

8 Cosgrove DM III, Heric B, Lytle BW, et al: Aprotinin therapy for reoperative myocardial revascularization: A placebo-controlled trial. Ann Thorac Surg 1992;54:1031–1038.
9 Del Rossi AJ, Cernaianu AC, Botros S, Lemole GM, Moore R: Prophylactic treatment of postperfusion bleeding using EACA. Chest 1989;96:27–30.
10 Helm RE, Rosengart TK, Klemperer JD, Gomez M, DeBois WJ, Gold JP, Ko W, Velasco F, Altorki N, Lang S, Thomas S, Isom OW, Krieger KH: Comprehensive multimodality blood conservation: 100 consecutive CABG operations without transfusion. Ann Thorac Surg 1998; 65:125–136.

Karl H. Krieger, MD, Department of Cardiothoracic Surgery,
The New York-Presbyterian Hospital-New York Weill Cornell Medical Center,
525 East 68th Street, New York, NY 10021 (USA)

Borer JS, Isom OW (eds): Pathophysiology, Evaluation and Management of Valvular Heart Diseases.
Adv Cardiol. Basel, Karger, 2002, vol 39, pp 184–188

Emerging Role of Complementary Medicine in Valvular Surgery

Mehmet Oz

Columbia University, College of Physicians and Surgeons, New York, N.Y., USA

This survey document should reveal valuable lessons that we have acquired over the past 5 years using alternative approaches to facilitate the recovery of patients undergoing heart surgery. We have found these approaches to be especially valuable for patients undergoing high-risk procedures, including many individuals requiring valvular surgery.

Complementary medicine is just as cutting edge for surgery as the use of robots. We should be incorporating innovative ways of healing patients that are equally ambitious and novel. Much of the battle towards integrative medicine is won if we can alter the different perspectives that patients and physicians bring to their relationship. I hope to review tools that we can incorporate into our day-to-day practice that can facilitate this process for a busy cardiac specialist.

Approximately 50% of patients incorporate alternative medicine into their lives even though they are healthy. Herbal therapies and chiropractic treatments are probably the two most common modalities next to religion. These observations prompted us to approach patients who enter a cardiac surgeons office and survey their use of alternative therapies. Approximately 70% respond affirmatively [1]. If you exclude vitamins and prayer, two therapies that many people do not really consider alternative, you are left with about 45% of patients using alternative therapies including herbs that may influence the peri-operative course of these patients [1, 2].

When we ask these patients if they asked or discussed with their heart surgeons any of these aspects of their well-being, only 20% report having even broached the issue with their physician. More importantly, even if prompted, only 37% of patients would share this information with their physician. We have a communication gap with our patient population, and we are encountering problems which might be avoidable. Table 1 includes a list of commonly used

Table 1. Common products and herbs that may affect surgical outcomes

Product	Effects
Coagulation	
Dehydroepiandrosterone (DHEA)	Interacts with plasminogen activator inhibitor and tissue plasminogen activator
Eicosapentaenoic acid (EPA)	Decreases platelet aggregation
Fish oils	Increase fibrinolysis
Garlic	Inhibits platelet aggregation
Onion	Inhibits platelet aggregation
Vitamin E	Inhibits platelet aggregation
Feverfew	Interacts with warfarin
Ginko biloba	Interacts with warfarin
Coenzyme Q_{10}	Interacts with warfarin
Ginger	Interacts with warfarin
Ginseng	Interacts with warfarin
St. John's wort	Interacts with warfarin
Hemodynamics	
Caffeine	Hypertension
Ephedra	Hypertension
Drug interactions	
Hawthorn berry	Interacts with digoxin
Licorice	Interacts with digoxin
Plaintain	Interacts with digoxin
Uzara root	Interacts with digoxin
Ginseng	Interacts with digoxin
St. John's wort	Interacts with digoxin, warfarin, oral contraceptives, cyclosporin, antiviral drugs
Iron	Affects bioavailability
Grapefruit	Cyclosporin

herbs and vitamins that interact with widely used conventional pharmaceuticals including digoxin and tissue plasminogen activator (tPA). Many of these products also alter platelet adhesion and fibrinolysis. At a very superficial level, restoring an open dialog with our patients is a critical issue for us to address as cardiovascular physicians.

There are also some more subtle aspects of the mind-body movement that we are beginning to study. For example, subjects in several studies have demonstrated that the highest incidence of myocardial infarctions is on Monday mornings [3]. We must address these putatively emotional issues as we try to improve the well-being of our patients.

Music is a good example of this effort. Many patients ask, 'Do audio tapes work in the operating room?' Most people would say, 'Probably not.' Patients rarely recall having open heart surgery, and most people do not have pain during open heart surgery. We also know patients cannot move because we can check for paralysis, and we know patients do not remember their procedures. But we do not know about awareness. We started this field of study by looking at the response to auditory-evoked potentials. We played clicks in patient ears, placed EEG leads on their heads, and looked at the early, mid and late evoked potentials. The middle latency period connotes awareness. In every studied patient, awareness was evident throughout the cardiac surgical procedure [4].

So then, we have to go to the second question. If patients are subconsciously aware during heart surgery, can I condition that awareness? We studied this problem using word pairs. Before the operation we asked each patient a series of word pairs and recorded the results. During surgery, they were subjected to audiotapes that either had no sound or had word pairs similar to the ones they heard in the pre-operative study. Five days later, they re-answered the word pair questions, but this time we noticed statistically significant differences in part predicted by the intra-operative tapes.

Now we are left with the third and most compelling question. If patients are aware during surgery and are susceptible to conditioning, can you condition awareness so the patient performance improves? Data from randomized study in spine surgery, a field which appears to have less surgeon-dependent bleeding, demonstrates statistically significant differences in bleeding based on which audiotapes were used by the patient group. Interestingly, in one group, use of audiotapes seemed to predispose to bleeding, once again cautioning us to recognize that any technique strong enough to help a patient is also powerful enough to hurt an individual. No effective therapy could possibly be deemed 100% safe.

We have also conducted a variety of studies evaluating different aromas and how they influence behavior. Humans use perfume to enhance different moods. On the other hand, patients walk into a hospital, smell the ammonia on the floor and get nauseated immediately. In order to study these smells in a stress setting, we needed to stimulate either emotional or physical stress, and we needed to access the patient's appropriate sense receptors. We asked patients to count back rapidly by 7 s, and during this stressful episode we exposed them to different aromas. Since aromatherapy is so poorly understood, we are forced to use relatively crude tools to identify subtle differences in how patients respond to these odors. For example, 15% of the population abhor scents that are adored by the remaining population. Once these subtleties are overcome, we can identify that aromas affect basic physiologic responses to stress such as the physiologic blood pressure and heart rate responses.

With a pure mind-body intervention-like guided imagery, we have been intrigued to find that in a randomized trial with 20 patients who are waiting for heart transplantation, participants felt subjectively better although their response to exercise testing demonstrated no objective benefits [5]. Physicians argue that the latter benefit is more important. Many patients might prefer a better quality of life, even if longevity is not prolonged. This modality may ideally demonstrate that complementary does not mean 'instead of' but rather 'together with' and improves our ability to customize treatment to our customers.

At New York-Presbyterian Hospital, we have a full-time massage therapist who teaches yoga classes as well. We have found intra- and peri-operative audiotapes relatively easy to provide to the patients. They are inexpensive and simple to use, so we subsidize their price and encourage patients to use the tapes whenever possible. Hospital food is a ubiquitous concern. Although we have been unable to measurably improve the quality of the diet, we have convinced the hospital to support free dried fruit and nuts which are distributed by our volunteer staff. They are easy to store, relatively inexpensive and provide the nurses a solution for patients who refuse to eat the hospital food. Finally, religion, which is the single most commonly reported 'alternative' technique used by patients, is underused in the modem hospital according to several surveys [6]. We ought to have a consultative relationship with our pastoral services so that we can use them as our allies in managing patients who are undergoing valve surgery and need support. Interestingly, most patients actually would prefer to speak to someone who is gifted in that area, rather than talking to the heart specialist.

Many of these integrated therapies address the physiological challenges that our patients bring us. As we increase our awareness of the importance of these issues to patient well-being, we will need to add a more diverse set of tools to our armamentarium to provide the best care possible. Much of this innovative work was done by psychiatry departments surveying our patients undergoing open-heart surgery. Approximately 20% have clinically diagnosable depression [7], and this cohort has a much higher incidence of post-operative complications compared to the non-depressed 80% of the population. Next to ejection fraction and female gender, depression appears to be one of the most important predictors of complications following acute myocardial infarction [8] and cardiac surgery. Living alone also has borderline significant impact and is linked to major depression. Optimistic patients are less likely to have infections and other major adverse cardiac complications [9]. Data from the Veterans Administration health care system [10] evaluating 6-month mortality following coronary artery bypass grafting reveals physical component summary score as a highly significant predictor with a risk ratio of 1.39 ($p = 0.006$) for cardiac events after open-heart surgery. In effect, we are learning that the patients' belief in their progress is an important predictor in addition to the physicians' assessment.

As our traditional treatment options for disease improve, we will need to push the envelop further to provide the best care for our patients. In some instances, this will require the use of innovative technologies to make procedures more palatable. Often, the battle can be advanced by using simpler treatments that many of our patients are already incorporating into their personal treatment programs. The physician community is obliged to evaluate, although not advocate, integrative approaches or we risk no longer being a valuable resource for patients in this arena.

References

1 Liu EH, Turner LM, Lin SX, Klaus L, Choi LY, Whitworth I, Ting W, Oz MC: Use of alternative medicine by patients undergoing cardiac surgery. J Thorac Cardiovasc Surg 2000;120:335–341.
2 Witte KA, Clark AL, Cleland JGF: Chronic heart failure and micronutrients. J Am Coll Cardiol 2001;37:1765–1774.
3 Muller JE, Stone PH, Turi ZG, Rutherford JD, Czeisler CA for the MILIS Study Group: Circadian variation in the frequency of onset of acute myocardial infarction. N Engl J Med 1985;313: 1315–1322.
4 Adams DC, Madigan JD, Hilton HJ, Szerlip NJ, Cooper LA, Emerson RG, Smith CR, Rose EA, Oz MC: Evidence for unconscious memory processing during elective cardiac surgery. Circulation 1998;98(suppl):289–293.
5 Klaus L, Beniaminovitz A, Choi L, Greenfield F, Whitworth GC, Oz MC, Mancini DM: Pilot study of guided imagery use in severe heart failure. Am J Cardiol 2000;86:101–104.
6 Harris WS, Gowda M, Kolb JW, Strychacz CP, Vacek JL, Jones PG, Forker A, O'Keefe JH, McCallister BD: A randomized, controlled trial of the effects of remote, intercessory prayer on outcomes in patients admitted to the coronary care unit. Arch Intern Med 1999;159:2273–2278.
7 Connerney I, Shapiro PA, McLaughlin JS, Bagiella E, Sloan RP: Relation between depression after coronary artery bypass surgery and 12-month outcome: A prospective study. Lancet 2001;358:1766–1771.
8 Frasure-Smith N, Lesperance F: Depression following myocardial infarction. JAMA 1993;270: 1819–1825.
9 Scheier MF, Matthews KA, Owens JF, Schulz R, Bridges MW, Macgovern GJ, Carver CS: Optimism and rehospitalization after coronary artery bypass graft surgery. Arch Intern Med 1999;159:829–835.
10 Rumsfeld JS, MaWhinney S, McCarthy M, Shroyer ALW, VillaNueva CB, O'Brien M, Moritz TE, Henderson WG, Grover FL, Sethi GK, Hammermeister KE: Health-related quality of life as a predictor of mortality following CABG surgery. JAMA 1999;281:1298–1303.

Mehmet Oz, MD, Columbia University, College of Physicians and Surgeons,
177 Ft. Washington Avenue, New York, NY 10032 (USA)

Borer JS, Isom OW (eds): Pathophysiology, Evaluation and Management of Valvular Heart Diseases.
Adv Cardiol. Basel, Karger, 2002, vol 39, pp 189–194

Factors Determining Selection of Valve Prosthesis – Tissue or Mechanical: Current Status

Subhasis Chatterjee, Timothy J. Gardner

Hospital of the University of Pennsylvania, Philadelphia, Pa., USA

The increasing prevalence of valvular heart disease combined with an aging population and improved cardiovascular surgical techniques have made heart valve surgery increasingly more common. One of the critical surgical decisions with such surgery remains the choice of the appropriate valve prosthesis. In this discussion, we review the relevant factors that determine whether a patient is more suitable for a mechanical or a bioprosthetic valve prosthesis and also evaluate the role of stentless xenografts and pulmonary auto-grafts.

The Society of Thoracic Surgeons (STS) Adult Cardiac Surgery Database reports approximately 130,000 aortic valve replacements (isolated AVR, AVR/CABG, and AVR/MVR) during 2000, with a risk-adjusted operative mortality of 4% for isolated AVR. In addition, there were approximately 75,000 mitral valve repairs/replacements (isolated MVR, MVR/CABG) with a risk-adjusted operative mortality of 7% for an isolated mitral valve replacement [1].

Since the 1960s, more than 80 different heart valve substitutes have been designed. The ideal prosthetic heart valve, however, still eludes development. Specifically, the perfect substitute heart valve would be durable and free from structural degeneration, thereby avoiding the need for risky re-operative surgery. Also, the ideal prosthesis would maintain an optimal hemodynamic profile characterized by central non-obstructive flow and without hemolysis. Finally, it would have a low rate of thromboembolism, thereby avoiding the need for systemic anticoagulation with its associated bleeding risks.

The two major types of currently used heart valves include mechanical and tissue prostheses. In general, the advantages of a mechanical prosthesis include excellent durability while the major disadvantage is the need for permanent anticoagulation. On the other hand, bioprosthetic valves do not require anticoagulation but have a limited durability, thought to be about 10–15 years, which subjects the younger patient to the need for re-operation. Table 1 displays the results of five studies comparing the complication rates associated with mechanical and bioprosthetic valves [2].

Examples of mechanical valves include the caged-ball Starr-Edwards valve, the single-tilting disk Medtronic-Hall and Omnicarbon valves, and the bileaflet-tilting disk valves such as the St. Jude Medical, Carbomedics, and Edwards-Duromedics valves. Examples of the bioprosthetic valves include allograft valves such as the Hancock Porcine, Carpentier-Edwards Porcine, Carpentier-Edwards Bovine Pericardial, and the Stentless Porcine valves. There are, as well, cryopreserved human homograft valves available currently.

At the present time, about two-thirds of patients receive mechanical valves. Current practice guidelines suggest that bioprosthetic valves are best suited for patients older than 70 years undergoing AVR because of the assumption that the patient's life expectancy is likely to be less than the lifespan of the bioprosthetic valve, making re-operation unlikely. In addition, in patients in whom there are specific contraindications to anticoagulation, i.e., women of childbearing age or patients in whom noncompliance with anticoagulation may be a concern, a bioprosthetic valve avoids the need for anticoagulation required for a mechanical valve. On the other hand, mechanical valves are recommended in younger patients (life expectancy >10 years), patients undergoing double valve procedures, or patients already anticoagulated for another reason, i.e., mitral valve replacement in a patient with chronic atrial fibrillation.

The current trends in valve surgery have resulted in the refinement of some of these traditional recommendations [3]. With respect to mechanical valves, there have been modifications in anticoagulation protocols with an acceptance of a lower level of anticoagulation (lower PT/INR) in an effort to reduce bleeding complications without a corresponding increase in thromboembolic complications. These improvements in anticoagulation outpatient regimens and the creation of dedicated anticoagulation clinics have insured better management of these patients and have prevented both over- and under-anticoagulation. Both bleeding and thromboembolism risks of mechanical valves have been reduced.

With respect to bioprosthetic valves, currently there are more elderly patients presenting with degenerative valve disease compared to fewer younger patients with rheumatic heart disease. Bioprosthetic valves can and are being more readily applied to this older group of patients. Moreover, the addition of anti-calcification agents to bioprosthetic valves has extended their lifespan, making re-operative valve surgery less likely in elderly patients. In addition, overall improvements in cardiac surgery techniques and myocardial protection have made re-operation safer. Thus, many patients in their 60s are offered bioprosthetic valves with the

Table 1. Comparison of complications in mechanical and bioprosthetic valves [from 2, with permission]

Complication	Peterseim, 1999 (NR)		Holper et al., 1995 (NR)		Myken et al., 1995 (NR)		Hammermeister et al., 1993 (R)		Bloomfield et al., 1991 (R)	
	bio (n = 429)	mech (n = 326)	bio (n = 326)	mech (n = 250)	bio (n = 100)	mech (n = 100)	bio (n = 126)	mech (n = 198)	bio (n = 102)	mech (n = 109)
Hemorrhage, %/patient-year	0.3	1.2	0.94	3.0	0.1	2.3	2.2	3.9	0.81	2.7
Thromboembolism	0.7	1.0	1.29	1.32	0.6	1.2	1.4	1.5	1.9	0.96
Leak, %/patient-year	0.7	1.0	0.14	0.24			0.18	0.36		
Endocarditis, %/patient-year	0.4	0.4	0.14	0.36	0.6	0.5	0.73	0.64	0.18	0.4

NR = Nonrandomized; R = randomized.

knowledge that subsequent re-operative surgery 10–15 years later may not be prohibitively risky.

In a comprehensive study assessing the risk of re-operative bioprosthetic valve replacements since 1986, Akins et al. [4] reviewed six published series consisting of over 2,000 MVR patients and 1,200 AVR patients. The average MVR death rate was 11.5% and ranged from 10.0 to 15.3% while the AVR death rate was 10.3% with a range of 9.8 to 11.5%. In Akins' series of 400 re-operative AVR and MVR for failed bioprostheses, they noted that the average age of the patient was 64 years, the mortality was 7.8%, and 27% had a prolonged length of stay. Multivariate predictors of mortality were age >65, male gender, renal insufficiency, and non-elective surgery. In elective first re-operative surgery, good results were observed with a 4.8% mortality (7/147). Thus, for the majority of patients with a bioprosthetic valve, re-operative surgery can be performed safely.

Moreover, the indications for bioprosthetic valve placement is further expanding with a better understanding of the natural history of other co-morbid medical conditions to subsequent lifespan. Peterseim et al. [5] studied the fate of bioprosthetic valves in such patients. They noted that in patients with significant co-morbid conditions, the actual 10-year life expectancy was reduced, making a bioprosthetic valve with a high degree of freedom from re-operation at 10 years a suitable alternative. Specifically, it was noted that valvular surgery candidates with renal insufficiency (any age), lung disease (age >60), LVEF <40% (any age), or CAD (any age) all have low 10-year survival rates ranging between 27 and 35%. Such patients have a correspondingly low re-operation rate at 10 years, ranging from 0 to 5%. Thus, in patients requiring valve replacement who have significant co-morbid conditions, a bioprosthetic valve is a reasonable choice given the shorter lifespan and low likelihood for re-operation, regardless of the patient's age.

Stentless porcine xenografts and aortic root homografts have been used for aortic valve replacement for many years. Although these procedures require more complex implantation techniques with longer ischemic and cardiopulmonary bypass (CPB) times, the hemodynamic characteristics of such valve substitutes are favorable and resemble those of native aortic valves. Stentless porcine bioprostheses are being used more commonly today based on a reduction in obstruction from stents, with a resultant reduction in tissue stresses and improved hemodynamic characteristics. There has been evidence to suggest a progressive increase in effective orifice area (EOA) and a decrease in transvalvular gradients as well as a normalization of LV mass index and wall thickness within 6–12 months. Examples include the porcine Medtronic Freestyle Stentless valve and the St. Jude Toronto Stentless Porcine valve (SPV).

Vrandecic et al. [6] compared the results of stented (n = 157) to stentless (n = 175) valves and found that the freedom from re-operation at 10 years in the stentless valve group was 98.9 ± 0.7% compared to 63.2 ± 13.4% in the stented group ($p < 0.05$). In addition, the stentless group also had a lower rate of overall complications (3.4 vs. 12%, $p < 0.05$) compared to the stented group. Although these results are encouraging, such findings have not been uniformly duplicated. Cohen et al. [7] noted in a multicenter randomized trial of 99 patients that there were no significant differences in hemodynamic indices or LV mass regression between patients with stented and stentless aortic valve prostheses at 12 months.

The pulmonary autograft, or Ross procedure, was first described by Donald Ross in 1967 for aortic valve replacement. It was postulated that the pulmonary autograft might function indefinitely with freedom from calcification, thromboembolism, and risk of bleeding. The autograft is felt to remain viable and actually grow in children, and a homograft with valve is placed in pulmonary position. This procedure, however, involving a complex double valve replacement, has had an increased initial morbidity and morality.

In Ross' series [8] of 241 patients from 1967 to 1986, the 30-day mortality rate was 6.6%, and 50% of patients maintained freedom from re-operation at 20 years. Jaggers et al. [9] compared the Ross procedure ($n = 22$) to mechanical AVRs ($n = 27$). They noted that, despite the longer operative time and more expensive pulmonary valve homograft compared to the mechanical valve, the cost savings from avoiding anticoagulation in the pulmonary autograft group made the procedures equivalent in cost (pulmonary autograft = USD 23,226 ± 6,960 vs. mechanical = USD 23,140 ± 7,825, p = NS). Moreover, there was a lower rate of significant valve complications in the PV autograft group (1/22, 5%) compared to the mechanical group (6/27, 22%, $p < 0.05$).

These encouraging reports of favorable hemodynamic outcomes with stentless porcine allograft prostheses for aortic valve replacement have resulted in increasing utilization of such valve substitutes. The use of the pulmonary autograft, however, appears to have declined somewhat in the last several years and is now used most commonly for children with aortic stenosis.

In summary, the vast majority of heart valve replacements today involve either mechanical or bioprosthetic valve substitutes. The increasing success of mitral valve repair procedures has reduced mitral valve replacement. The most commonly replaced valve is the aortic. Freedom from structural degeneration of current bioprostheses is reduced especially in patients >65 years who require aortic valve replacement. The currently available bi-leaflet mechanical prostheses require less anticoagulation to avoid thromboembolic complications. The cryopreserved homograft valves are particularly useful in patients with endocarditis. The non-stented porcine allograft valves may reduce prosthesis-induced residual transvalvular gradients. The pulmonary autograft aortic valve replacement is effective in patients with small aortic roots, especially children with aortic stenosis.

References

1 www.sts.org – Society of Thoracic Surgeons Database.
2 Vongpatansin W, Hillis DL, Lange RA: Medical progress: Prosthetic heart valves. N Engl J Med 1996;335:407–416.
3 Birkmeyer NJO, Birkmeyer JD, Tosteson ANA, et al: Prosthetic valve type for patients undergoing aortic valve replacement: A decision analysis. Ann Thorac Surg 2000;70:1946–1952.
4 Akins CW, Buckley MJ, Daggett WM, et al: Risk of reoperative valve replacement for failed mitral and aortic valve prostheses. Ann Thorac Surg 1998;65:1545–1552.
5 Peterseim DS, Cen YY, Cheruvu S, et al: Long-term outcome after biologic versus mechanical aortic valve replacement in 841 patients. J Thorac Cardiovasc Surg 1999;117:890–897.
6 Vrandecic M, Fantini FA, Filho BG, et al: Retrospective clinical analysis of stented vs. stentless porcine aortic bioprostheses. Eur J Cardiothorac Surg 2000;18:46–53.
7 Cohen G, Christakis GT, et al: Are stentless valves hemodynamically superior to stented valves? A prospective randomized trial. Ann Thorac Surg 2002;73:767–778.
8 Matsuki O, Okta Y, Almeida RS, et al: Two decades experience with aortic valve replacement with pulmonary autograft. J Thorac Cardiovasc Surg 1988;95:705–711.
9 Jaggers J, Harrison JK, Bashore TM, et al: The Ross procedure: Shorter hospital stay, decreased morbidity, and cost effective. Ann Thorac Surg 1998;65:1553–1557.

Timothy J. Gardner, MD, FACS, Hospital of the University of Pennsylvania,
3400 Spruce Street, Silverstein 6, Philadelphia, PA 19104 (USA)
Tel. +1 215 6622022, Fax +1 215 3495798

Borer JS, Isom OW (eds): Pathophysiology, Evaluation and Management of Valvular Heart Diseases.
Adv Cardiol. Basel, Karger, 2002, vol 39, pp 195–202

Selective Aspects of Infective Endocarditis: Considerations on Diagnosis, Risk Factors, Treatment and Prophylaxis

Barry Jay Hartman

New York Presbyterian Hospital-New York Weill Cornell Medical Center,
New York, N.Y., USA

Infective endocarditis is an infection that involves the heart valves primarily. It is not a common infection, occurring in only about 1 patient per 1,000 admissions in the United States with the average age of the patient being about 50 years. There are several major risk factors that predispose to valves becoming infected. These include congenital heart disease, rheumatic heart disease, degenerative heart disease, intravenous drug usage, the presence of prosthetic valves, mitral valve prolapse, and indwelling intravenous catheters.

Prior to the development of antibiotics, this infection had a mortality rate approximating 100%. Nonetheless, since antibiotics, the mortality rate has been considerably reduced. However, the infection can lead to significant valvular destruction and valvular dysfunction often requiring valve replacement even when the infection itself has been eradicated.

In this paper, I will discuss four specific aspects of endocarditis. The first will be the new criteria for defining and diagnosing infective endocarditis. The second part of the discussion will be on intravascular device-associated endocarditis primarily from *Staphylococcus aureus* which now accounts for 20–30% of all cases of endocarditis. The third discussion will revolve around short-course treatments for viridans streptococcal endocarditis. Lastly, I will discuss some future considerations related to antibiotic prophylaxis to prevent infective endocarditis.

Diagnosis

It is not always obvious or easy to diagnose infective endocarditis. The most common organisms that cause endocarditis, viridans streptococci, can also be organisms that are frequent contaminants in blood culture bottles either from the skin of the patient or from the laboratory itself. Therefore, the presence of the organism in the blood does not always mean infective endocarditis. In 1981, Von Reyn and associates proposed a definition of endocarditis based on what was referred to as a 'strict case definition'. However, these criteria were not all-inclusive and in 1994, Durack et al. [1] proposed a new group of guidelines and criteria (Duke criteria) for diagnosing infective endocarditis that now included echocardiographic findings to improve the specificity of the diagnostic criteria. The Duke criteria were modified in 1997 [2], and have been proven to be highly specific in several studies (table 1). The 'definitive criteria' of endocarditis include a pathological diagnosis by culture of the vegetation at the time of surgery and by the presence of the vegetation seen under the microscope by the pathologist. In those cases in which the valve cannot be obtained, 'clinical criteria' are used to make the diagnosis that include *major criteria* such as positive blood cultures from typical organisms that cause endocarditis particularly when the cultures are multiple or persistently positive. In addition, evidence of valvular involvement by echocardiography showing a vegetation, abscess, dehiscence of a prosthetic valve, or new valvular insufficiency are major criteria that could be used for the diagnosis of endocarditis. A set of *minor criteria* include the presence of fever, underlying heart disease, various types of embolic or immune related phenomena as well as less specific echocardiographic and microbiologic diagnoses. Recently, additional minor criteria such as splenomegaly, elevated erythrocyte sedimentation rate, high C-reactive protein, etc., were added to the list. Using the Duke criteria, the specificity is as high as 99%, confirming the utility of this particular modality.

The importance of having an accurate diagnosis for infective endocarditis is that treatment is dependent on that diagnosis. For those patients who have a bacteremia without infective endocarditis, therapy is generally 10–14 days. However, in those patients that have infective endocarditis, the therapy, depending on the organism, can be extended to 4–6 weeks usually with intravenous therapy, thereby increasing cost and inconvenience to the patient. In addition, uniformity of diagnosis allows the results of studies on various aspects of infective endocarditis to be more accurate and relevant.

Intravascular Device-Associated Endocarditis

The National Nosocomial Surveillance Infection Survey has shown that over the past 30 years the incidence of *S. aureus* bacteremia has increased 250–300% in the hospital and outpatient settings. Much of this can be attributed to the use of indwelling catheters and other intravascular devices that increase the risk for *S. aureus* bacteremia. Though *S. aureus* accounts for only 20–30% of all cases of endocarditis, it accounts for the majority of cases of intravascular device-associated endocarditis. In fact, 50% of all *S. aureus* endocarditis is now

Table 1. Diagnosis of infective endocarditis (Duke and modified Duke criteria) [from 1, 2, with permission]

Definitive infective endocarditis

Pathologic criteria

- Microorganisms: cultures or histology in a vegetation
- Pathologic lesions: vegetation or intracardiac abscess

Clinical criteria

- 2 major criteria
- 1 major and 3 minor criteria
- 5 minor criteria

Possible infective endocarditis

- Findings consistent with, but fall short of, definitive, but not rejected

Rejected infective endocarditis

- Firm alternate diagnosis
- Resolution of endocarditis syndrome with antibiotics for 4 days or less
- No pathologic evidence at surgery or autopsy, after antibiotics for 4 days or less

---

Major criteria

Positive blood cultures

- Typical microorganisms
- Persistently positive blood cultures with organisms consistent with endocarditis
  - Blood cultures drawn over 12 h apart
  - All of 3, or majority of 4 or more separate cultures drawn at least 1 h apart

Evidence of endocardial involvement

- Positive echocardiogram for infective endocarditis with 'vegetation', abscess; new partial dehiscence of prosthetic valve; or new valvular regurgitation

Minor criteria

- Predisposition: Predisposing heart conditon
- Fever: $>$ 38°C
- Vascular phenomenon: Arterial emboli; septic pulmonary infarcts; mycotic aneurysm, intracranial hemorrhage, Janeway lesions
- Immunologic phenomenon: Glomerulonephritis; Osler nodes; Roth spots, rheumatoid factor
- Echocardiogram: Consistent with infective endocarditis but not meeting major criteria
- Microbiologic evidence: Positive blood culture but not meeting major criteria or positive serologic evidence of active infection consistent with infective endocarditis

Additional minor criteria

- New splenomegaly
- New clubbing
- Splinter hemorrhages
- Petechiae
- High ESR ($>$ 30 mm/h if age $<$ 60 years; $>$ 50 mm/h if age $>$ 60 years)
- High C-reactive protein $>$ 100 mg/l
- Microscopic hematuria
- Central nonfeeding venous lines
- Peripheral venous lines

secondary to intravascular devices. Some of these patients respond quickly to removing the intravascular device and prompt initiation of antibiotic treatment, but on occasion if only a short course of treatment is given, the patient returns several weeks later with severe valvular involvement or some major embolic event secondary to endocarditis that was missed and improperly treated at the time of the patient's bacteremia. A recent study [3] done at Duke University looked prospectively at 59 patients who had infective endocarditis due to *S. aureus*. The authors divided the infections into hospital-acquired or community-acquired. In this group of 59 patients, Duke criteria were used to determine if there was endocarditis. When one looks at both groups of patients, 39% of the patients, whether they were in or out of the hospital, had intravascular catheters and another 12% had renal dialysis grafts, fistulas or catheters. Therefore, for 50% of the patients, whether community-acquired or hospital-acquired, the *S. aureus* bacteremia was associated in some way with an intravascular catheter. This study also evaluated results of transthoracic echocardiography and transesophageal echocardiography and showed that only 34% of the patients had evidence of endocarditis by transthoracic echocardiography, but 85% had evidence by transesophageal echocardiography. If abscesses were present, all were found by the transesophageal echocardiogram. The overall death rate was 22% in both groups, consistent with the high mortality reported from *S. aureus* endocarditis, particularly in the elderly.

From this study and others [4], it appears that between 20 and 25% of patients who have *S. aureus* bacteremia actually develop endocarditis. This means that almost 1 in 4 patients should require prolonged courses of antibiotics rather than 10–14 days. Because of this high percentage, it might be reasonable to give all patients with *S. aureus* bacteremia a prolonged course of 4–6 weeks of treatment, but this would be expensive and have potential complications from treatment and the intravascular devices used for the treatment. As suggested by others, one could obtain a transesophageal echocardiogram on patients with *S. aureus* bacteremia and if there is definitive evidence of endocarditis, a prolonged course of treatment could be given. If the echocardiogram was negative, one could consider a short course of treatment, assuming there was no other evidence of endocarditis. At this point there are no formal recommendations to deal with patients who have *S. aureus* bacteremia from intravascular devices, but this may be one approach for many patients.

Short-Course Therapy for Infective Endocarditis

One of the main treatment characteristics of infective endocarditis has been the need for a prolonged course of 4–6 weeks, often with multiple antibiotics. Over the years, easier courses of treatment have been used in specific settings.

Table 2. Short-course treatments for penicillin-susceptible viridens streptococcal endocarditis[1] [from 5, with permission]

Microbiological outcome	Monotherapy recipients[2] (n = 23)		Combination therapy recipients[3] (n = 23)	
	n	%	n	%
Cure	22	95.7	22	95.7
Reinfection	1	4.3	0	
Treatment failure	0		1	4.3

[1] Microbiological outcome for 46 patients with endocarditis due to penicillin-susceptible streptococci who were treated with monotherapy with ceftriaxone 2g. i.v. daily for 4 weeks or combination therapy with ceftriaxone 2 g i.v. daily plus gentamicin 3 mg/kg once daily for 2 weeks.

[2] Three patients in this group were not evaluable for microbiological outcome.

[3] Two patients in this group were not evaluable for microbiological outcome.

Several years ago, studies from Switzerland and elsewhere showed that, for sensitive strains of viridans streptococcal endocarditis, ceftriaxone 2 g intravenously daily for a period of 4 weeks was equal to multiple doses of penicillin with or without an aminoglycoside for the same period of time. The advantage of the former regimen was that only one antibiotic was given once daily, allowing for simplification of home intravenous antibiotic therapy. This still required 4 weeks of treatment. In a more recent study, however, ceftriaxone 2 g intravenously daily for 4 weeks was compared to ceftriaxone plus gentamicin each given once daily for a total duration of only 2 weeks [5] (table 2). The results were similar in both groups. However, after the combination therapy for 2 weeks, there was a considerably higher number of patients that eventually had to have surgery for cure, but this did not reach statistical significance. At this time, I cannot recommend this two week regimen for all patients until more studies confirm that this is an equal regimen without added toxicity. We might reserve this for younger patients with normal kidney function and in those patients who would be unable to take treatment for 4 weeks or longer. This particular short regimen has not been shown to be effective for any other form of endocarditis than that due to viridans streptococci.

Prophylaxis

There has never been a controlled study in humans proving the benefit of antibiotic prophylaxis in the prevention of infective endocarditis. However, there have been animal models that have shown that prophylaxis can prevent experimentally induced endocarditis. It seems reasonable that this same approach should be effective in humans, particularly in those patients with risks of endocarditis. Over the years, consensus groups of infectious disease specialists and cardiologists have gotten together to make formal recommendations on prophylactic regimens to be used for specific valvular heart disease and for specific procedures being done to patients. These regimens and recommendations have changed slightly over the years with the last major change being in 1997 [9]. However, a question persists as to whether everybody in various risk groups should continue to use these regimens because we are particularly concerned about the inappropriate use of antibiotics and the development of bacterial resistance.

Everyone has short periods of bacteremia during the day from various routine activities and procedures such as brushing teeth, moving bowels, etc., and various procedures done by physicians or dentists carry known risk of bacteremia. It is based on these percentages that recommendations for antibiotic prophylaxis have evolved. Fortunately, even without antibiotic prophylaxis, the chance of getting endocarditis is relatively low (even with high-risk valvular heart disease or prosthetic valve replacements).

In an English study [6] that looked at the correlation between dental procedures and endocarditis, difficulty was found in correlating a specific risk. There are specific high-risk dental procedures, however, that seem to have a relatively high incidence of bacteremia and a greater risk for causing disease. These include extractions of the teeth, periodontal surgery, gingival surgery and various types of implantations.

In 1998, Strom et al. [7] (table 3) in Philadelphia looked at a population-based, case-control study of 273 patients. The study asked whether dental treatment was a risk factor for endocarditis by comparing a group of patients that had endocarditis with controls who were exactly the same age and had the same zip code who underwent the same number of dental procedures. Incidentally, most of these patients, in both groups, did not receive antibiotic prophylaxis. Therefore, this study could actually look at the risk and see whether or not there was a benefit for prophylaxis. As in the earlier English study, this study also showed that dental treatment did not seem to affect risk. However, if you had valve abnormalities, you had a higher risk of endocarditis regardless of whether you had dental procedures or not in the prior 3 months. The authors concluded that only a few cases of infective endocarditis could be prevented by dental prophylaxis even it were 100% protective. As we know, prophylaxis is not 100% protective and we would only be preventing approximately 2 cases per 1 million person-years if we gave all at-risk patients antibiotic prophylaxis for dental procedures. In addition, only 6 of 273 patients with endocarditis had tooth extractions within

Table 3. To prophylax or not to prophylax for dental procedures

1. Strom et al. [7]
   Population-based, case-control study of 273 patients

   Results: Dental treatment does not seem to be a risk factor for endocarditis
   Cardiac valvular abnormalities are strong risk factors

   Conclusion: Only a few cases of infective endocarditis could be prevented by dental prophylaxis even if it were 100% effective (~2 cases per 1,000,000 person-years)

2. Editorial by Durack [8]

   Assessment of Strom et al. study: 6/273 patients with endocarditis had tooth extractions within 2 months compared to 0/273 controls
   (p = NS; but possible type II error due to a few cases)

   Suggestions: Consider prophylaxis with 4 high risk factors:
   Dental extractions
   Gingival surgery or implant placement
   Prosthetic valves
   Previous endocarditis

   Results of suggestions: 80% benefits retained at 20% of the costs
   Reduced antibiotic resistance through reduced usage

2 months. Overall, that risk was relatively low, raising concern as to whether all at-risk patients should get antibiotics for the very few cases that might occur. The authors concluded that one should consider particular patients for prophylaxis when they undergo specific high-risk procedures such as dental extraction or gingival surgery or in those who are at very high risk from prosthetic valves or previous endocarditis. If you give prophylaxis to only those four groups of patients, you would obtain an 80% benefit at about 20% of the cost that we now have for giving it to all patients who have any risk from any procedure [8].

Despite these results, there has been no change in the recommendations of the American Heart Association (AHA) for antibiotic prophylaxis for endocarditis [9]. Personally, I would follow the AHA recommendations until and unless they are changed formally.

References

1 Durack DT, Lukes AS, Bright DK: The Duke Endocarditis Service. New criteria for diagnosis of infective endocarditis: Utilization of specific echocardiographic findings. Am J Med 1994;96: 200–209.

2 Lamas CC, Eykyn SJ: Suggested modifications to the Duke criteria for the clinical diagnosis of native valve and prosthetic valve endocarditis: Analysis of 118 pathologically proven cases. Clin Infect Dis 1977;25:713–719.

3 Fowler VG, Sanders LL, Kong LK, et al: Infective endocarditis due to *Staphylococcus aureus*: 59 prospectively identified cases with follow-up. Clin Infect Dis 1999;28:706–714.
4 Watanakunakorn C: Increasing importance of intravascular device-associated *Staphylococcus aureus* endocarditis. Clin Infect Dis 1999;28:115–116.
5 Sexten DJ, Tenenbaum MJ, Wilbon WR, et al: Ceftriaxone once daily for four weeks – compared to ceftriaxone plus gentamicin – once daily for two weeks for treatment of endocarditis due to penicillin-susceptible streptococci. Clin Infect Dis 1998;27:1470–1474.
6 Hall G, Hermdahl A, Nord CE: Bacteremia after oral surgery and antibiotic prophylaxis for endocarditis. Clin Infect Dis 1999;29:1–10.
7 Strom BL, Abrutyn E, Berlin JA, et al: Dental and cardiac risk factors for infective endocarditis – A population-based, case-control study. Ann Intern Med 1998;129:761–769.
8 Durack DT: Antibiotics for prevention of endocarditis during dentistry: Time to scale back? Ann Intern Med 1998;129:829–831.
9 Dajani AS, Taubert KA, Wilson W, Bolger AF, Bayer A, Ferrieri P, Gewitz MH, Shulman ST, Nouri S, Newburger JW, Hutto C, Pallasch TJ, Gage TW, Levison ME, Peter G, Zuccaro G Jr: Prevention of bacterial endocarditis. Recommendations by the American Heart Association. Circulation 1997;96:358–366.

Barry J. Hartman, MD, Infectious Diseases and Internal Medicine,
407 East 70th street, New York, NY 10021 (USA)

Borer JS, Isom OW (eds): Pathophysiology, Evaluation and Management of Valvular Heart Diseases.
Adv Cardiol. Basel, Karger, 2002, vol 39, pp 203–209

Echocardiographic Assessment of the Vegetation: Are There Characteristics that Mandate Prophylactic Surgical Intervention?

Marvin Berger

The Heart Institute, Beth Israel Medical Center New York, Department of Medicine, Albert Einstein College of Medicine, Bronx, N.Y., USA

Echocardiography plays an essential role in the diagnosis and management of infective endocarditis (IE) and its complications. At the present time, it is the only noninvasive technique available for direct visualization of vegetations. The earliest reports describing the use of echocardiography to detect vegetations appeared in the early 1970s and were based on M-mode echocardiography. Two-dimensional echocardiography, which became available several years later, increased the diagnostic accuracy of echocardiography by providing superior spatial resolution and allowing assessment of vegetation size, mobility and texture. More recently, the introduction of transesophageal echocardiography (TEE), has further improved the ability to visualize vegetations and abscesses. Studies in which the sensitivity of transthoracic echocardiography (TTE) and TEE were directly compared, TEE has consistently been superior in detecting vegetations on native [1–8] and prosthetic valves [3, 7, 9, 10] and in the identification of perivalvular abscesses [11, 12] (table 1).

Echocardiography and Prognosis

In addition to its role in the diagnosis of IE, echocardiography can provide important information about outcome. Patients with IE who have vegetations detected by echocardiography are at increased risk for embolic events, congestive heart failure, urgent surgery and death compared to those in whom vegetations

Table 1. Comparison of TTE and TEE in the detection of valvular vegetations, prosthetic valve endocarditis, and perivalvular abscess based on pooled data from multiple studies

	Patients, n	TTE sensitivity, %	TEE sensitivity, %
Vegetations	266	48	90
Prosthetic valve endocarditis	74	24	78
Perivalvular abscess	153	33	82

are not detected [13]. Vegetation characteristics such as size, mobility, texture, extent and location may also be helpful in predicting complications [14]. For example, large vegetations are more frequently associated with clinical complications than small vegetations. In a meta-analysis which included 738 patients from ten studies, large vegetations (>10 mm) were associated with a higher complication rate than small (>10 mm) or no vegetations [15]. The presence of a large vegetation was associated with an odds ratio of 2.95 for requiring valve replacement and 2.8 for increased risk of systemic embolization.

Embolic Events

Embolic events occur in 22–50% of patients with IE and are associated with significant morbidity and mortality. They may occur at any time in the course of the illness, but are most common during the first 2–4 weeks of treatment. Although certain echocardiographic findings have been associated with an increased embolic rate, determining the risk in an individual patient is extremely difficult. Numerous echocardiographic studies have been performed to determine if there are vegetation characteristics that are predictive of embolization in order to identify patients who might benefit from early surgery. Vegetation size and mobility are among the most frequently studied echocardiographic predictors of systemic embolization. Pooled data from several studies [2, 16, 17] show an embolic rate of 49% in patients with mobile or pedunculated vegetations, compared to 22% in patients with nonmobile vegetations (table 2). Studies assessing the predictive value of vegetation size have yielded conflicting results. Di Salvo et al. [17] performed TEE in 178 patients with definite IE based on the Duke criteria. The incidence of emboli was 60% in patients with vegetations >10 mm, and 70% in patients with vegetations >15 mm. Patients with severely mobile vegetations >15 mm were at the highest risk with an embolic rate of 83%. The authors concluded that vegetation morphology on TEE is helpful in predicting embolic

Table 2. Vegetation mobility and the frequency of embolic events

Author, year	Total patients	Frequency of embolic events with mobile or pedunculated vegetations	Frequency of embolic events with nonmobile or sessile vegetations	p value
Mügge, 1989	105	26/68 (38%)	7/37 (19%)	<0.001
Di Castro, 1997	57	21/46 (46%)	4/11 (36%)	NS
Di Salvo, 2001	178	45/73 (62%)	21/105 (20%)	<0.001
Total	349	92/187 (49%)	32/153 (21%)	<0.001

Table 3. Vegetation size and the frequency of embolic events

Author, year	Total patients	Frequency of embolic events with no vegetation or small vegetation (<10 mm)	Frequency of embolic events with large vegetation (>10 mm)	p value
Wong, 1983	31	3/15 (20%)	3/16 (19%)	NS
Lutas, 1986	76	8/50 (16%)	9/26 (35%)	NS
Buda, 1986	42	10/31 (32%)	6/11 (55%)	NS
Erbel, 1988	82	8/68 (12%)	3/14 (21%)	NS
Mügge, 1989	105	11/58 (19%)	22/47 (47%)	<0.01
Jaffe, 1990	50	2/18 (11%)	8/32 (25%)	NS
De Castro, 1997	57	9/19 (47%)	16/38 (42%)	NS
De Salvo, 2001	178	26/111 (23%)	40/67 (60%)	<0.001
Total	621	77/370 (21%)	107/251 (43%)	<0.001

events and may be of value in selecting patients for early surgical intervention. Sanfilippo et al. [14], using a logistic regression model to analyze the echocardiographic appearance of vegetations on TTE, also found that vegetation size and mobility were significant univariate predictors of emboli. Similar findings have been reported by others [18]. In contrast, Steckelberg et al. [19] studied 207 patients with TTE and found no relationship between vegetation size and embolic events. The findings in eight studies which examined the relationship between vegetation size and embolic events are summarized in table 3. Six of the eight studies showed an increased rate of embolization in patients with vegetations >10 mm. However in only two studies did the findings achieve statistical significance. When the data were pooled [13, 16, 17], the embolic rate was 43% patients with large vegetations (>10 mm) compared to 21% in patients with small (<10 mm) or no vegetations ($p < 0.01$). The failure of some studies to demonstrate a relationship between vegetation size and embolic events appears to be the result of low estatistical power due to a small sample size [15]. However, there are other factors involved such as poor standardization of diagnostic criteria for IE, the inclusion of patients with prosthetic valves, the use of TTE in some studies and TEE in others, and the inclusion of patients in whom the echocardiogram was obtained after the embolic event had already occurred. Therefore, although vegetation size and mobility appear to be associated with an increased incidence of embolic episodes, caution should be exerted in using vegetation morphology as the sole determinant in clinical decision-making.

There are additional factors beside vegetation size and mobility which may also influence the likelihood of embolic events. Mitral vegetations, especially those on the anterior leaflet, have a higher rate of embolization (25%) than the aortic vegetations (10%). There are certain infecting organisms such as staphylococcus and fungi, that are at high risk for embolization independent of vegetation size, whereas with staphylococcal infections, large vegetations are more likely to embolize than small vegetations.

Other Echocardiographic Characteristics That May Be Predictive of Outcome

As noted earlier, TEE is extremely useful for detecting perivalvular extension of IE. The detection of a perivalvular abscess is associated with increased mortality, more frequent development of congestive heart failure, and the need for surgical intervention. While an occasional patient with extension of the infection beyond the annulus may be successfully treated medically, the vast majority require operative intervention. There are also additional echocardiographic findings related to vegetation morphology and valve integrity that may be associated with clinical complications or an adverse outcome [14]. The presence of multiple vegetations or involvement of more than one leaflet may indicate a worse prognosis. Vegetations that are highly echogenic may indicate healing and appear to be associated with a lower complication rate. Valve perforation, which is best detected by color flow Doppler, is associated an increased incidence of congestive heart failure and frequently requires early surgical intervention. An increase in vegetation size over the course of therapy may identify a subset of patients with an increased rate of complications.

Right-Sided Endocarditis

Endocarditis involving right-sided cardiac valves occurs most commonly in intravenous drug users. In general, patients with right-sided endocarditis tend to have a lower mortality and are less likely to require surgery than patients with left-sided involvement. Vegetation size appears to be the most important echocardiographic predictor of outcome in patients with right-sided endocarditis. Although earlier studies suggested that vegetations >10 mm were associated with an adverse outcome, more recent work does not support this observation. Hecht and Berger [20] found a significant relationship between vegetation size and mortality in a study of 102 episodes of right-sided endocarditis. The mortality was 0% in patients with vegetations <10 mm, 2% in patients with vegetations 11–20 mm, and 33% in patients with vegetations >20 mm. Therefore, while large vegetations may be predictive of a poor outcome in right-sided endocarditis, the cut-off value appears to be higher than with left-sided involvement.

Endocarditis Related to Pacemaker Leads

Vegetations may also occur at other sites beside cardiac valves. Endocarditis related to pacemaker lead infection is an uncommon but serious complication of permanent transvenous pacing with a reported incidence of 0.13–7%. TEE appears to be extremely sensitive for detecting pacemaker lead-related endocarditis. In a recent study [21], TEE detected vegetations in 48 of 52 patients (92%) with pacemaker wire infections. Patients with this complication require removal of the entire pacing system. Vegetations <10 mm can be removed percutaneously, whereas vegetations ⩾10 mm usually require surgical removal.

Conclusions

Echocardiography, both TTE and TEE play an essential role in the diagnosis and management of IE. TEE is highly sensitive for the detection of vegetations and is especially useful in prosthetic valve endocarditis and for the detection of abscesses. Vegetation characteristics including size, mobility, texture and extent appear to be useful in identifying high-risk patients. In particular, large mobile vegetations localized to the anterior mitral leaflet pose a significant increased risk of embolization and it has been suggested by some that early surgery may be beneficial in these patients. Nevertheless, at the present time, there is still uncertainty as to whether surgical intervention based solely on vegetation morphology will improve outcome. There are however certain echocardiographic findings such as extension of infection beyond the annulus, severe valvular regurgitation in conjunction with congestive heart failure, and the presence of a vegetation on a pacemaker wire that almost invariably require surgical intervention. Right-sided endocarditis has a much better prognosis than left-sided endocarditis and in most cases can be managed medically, even when large vegetations are present. It is likely that advances in ultrasound technology and the accumulation of additional clinical data will further refine the role of echocardiography in the diagnosis and management of endocarditis and its complications.

References

1 Erbel R, Rohmann M, Drexler S, Mohr-Kahaly S, Gerharz CD, Iversen S, Oelert H, Meyer J: Improved diagnostic value of echocardiography in patients with infective endocarditis by transesophageal approach: A prospective study. Eur Heart J 1988;9:43–53.

2 Mugge A, Daniel WG, Gunter F, Lichtlen PR: Echocardiography in endocarditis: Reassessment of prognostic implications of vegetation size determined by the transthoracic and transesophageal approach. J Am Coll Cardiol 1989;14:631–638.

3 Taams MA, Gussenhoven EJ, Bos E, de Jaegere P, Roelandt JR, Sutherland GR, Bom N: Enhanced morphologic diagnosis in infective endocarditis by transesophageal echocardiography. Br Heart J 1990;63:109–113.

4 Shively B, Gurule FT, Roldan CA, Leggett JH, Schiller N: Diagnostic value of transesophageal compared with transthoracic echocardiography in infective endocarditis. J Am Coll Cardiol 1991;18:391–397.

5 Pedersen WR, Walker M, Olson JD, Gobel F, Lange HW, Daniel JA, Rogers J, Longe T, Kane M, Mooney MR, Goldenberg IF: Value of transesophageal echocardiography as an adjunct to transthoracic echocardiography in evaluation of native and prosthetic valve endocarditis. Chest 1991;100:351–356.

6 Birmingham GD, Rahko PS, Ballantyne F: Improved detection of infective endocarditis with transesophageal echocardiography. Am Heart J 1992;123:774–781.

7 Shapiro SS, Young E, De Guzman S, Ward J, Chiu C, Ginzton LE, Bayer AS: Transesophageal echocardiography in diagnosis of infective endocarditis. Chest 1994;105:377–382.

8 Lowry RW, Zoghbi WA, Baker WB, Wray RA, Quiñones MA: Clinical impact of transesophageal echocardiography in the diagnosis and management of infective endocarditis. Am J Cardiol 1994;73:1089–1091.

9 Khandheria BK, Seward JB, Oh JK, Freeman WK, Nichols BK, Sinak LJ, Miller FA, Tajik AJ: Value and limitations of transesophageal echocardiography in assessment of mitral valve prosthesis. Circulation 1991;83:1956–1968.

10 Daniel WG, Mugge A, Grote J, Hausmann D, Nikutta P, Laas J, Lichtlen PR, Martin RP: Comparison of transthoracic and transesophageal echocardiography for detection of abnormalities of prosthetic and bioprosthetic valves in the mitral and aortic positions. Am J Cardiol 1993;71:210–215.

11 Daniel WG, Mugge A, Martin RP, Lindert O, Hausmann D, Nonnast-Daniel B, Laas J, Lichtlen PR: Improvement in the diagnosis of abscesses associated with endocarditis by transesophageal echocardiography. N Engl J Med 1991;324:795–800.

12 Choussat R, Thomas D, Isnard TR, Michel PL, Iung B, Hanania G, Mathieu P, David M, du Roy de Chaumaray T, De Gevigney G, Le Breton H, Logeais Y, Pierre-Justin E, de Riberolles C, Morvan Y, Bischoff N: Perivalvular abscesses associated with endocarditis: Clinical features and prognostic factors of overall survival in a series of 233 cases. Eur Heart J 1999;20:232–241.

13 Mugge A, Daniel W: Echocardiographic assessment of vegetations in patients with infective endocarditis: Prognostic implications. Echocardiography 1995;12:651–661.

14 Sanfilippo AJ, Picard M, Newell JB, Rosas E, Davidoff R, Thomas JD, Weyman AE: Echocardiographic assessment of patients with infectious endocarditis: Prediction of risk for complications. J Am Coll Cardiol 1991;18:1191–1199.

15 Tischler M, Vaitkus PT: The ability of vegetation size on echocardiography to predict clinical complications: A meta-analysis. J Am Soc Echocardiogr 1997;10:62–68.

16 De Castro S, Magni G, Beni S, Cartoni D, Fiorelli M, Venditti M, Schwartz SL, Fedele F, Pandian NG: Role of transthoracic and transesophegeal echocardiography in predicting embolic events in patients with active endocarditis in involving native cardiac valves. Am J Cardiol 1997;80:1030–1034.
17 Di Salvo G, Habib G, Pergola V, Avierinos J, Philip E, Casalta J, Viailloud J, Derumeaux G, Gouvernet J, Ambrosi P, Lambert M, Ferracci A, Roualt D, Luccioni R: Echocardiography predicts embolic events in endocarditis. J Am Coll Cardiol 2001;37:1069–1076.
18 Stafford WJ, Petch J, Radford DJ: Vegetations in infective endocarditis: Clinical relevance and diagnosis by cross-sectional echocardiography. Br Heart J 1985;53:310–313.
19 Steckelberg JM, Murphy JG, Ballard D, Bailey K, Tajik AJ, Taliercio CP, Giuliani ER, Wilson WR: Emboli in infective endocarditis: The prognostic value of echocardiography. Ann Intern Med 1991;114:635–640.
20 Hecht SR, Berger M: Right-sided endocarditis in intravenous drug users. Prognostic features in 102 episodes. Ann Intern Med 1992;117:560–566.
21 Klug D, Lacroiz D, Savoye C, Goullard L, Grandmougin DL, Hennequin JL, Kacet S, Lekieffre J: Systemic infection related to endocarditis on pacemaker leads. Clinical presentation and management. Circulation 1997;95:2098–2107.

Marvin Berger, MD, Beth Israel Medical Center – 4 Silver,
First Avenue at 16th Street, New York, NY 10003 (USA)
E-Mail mberger@bethisraelny.org

Author Index

Subject Index